Does it hurt
when I press here two?

willgmblack

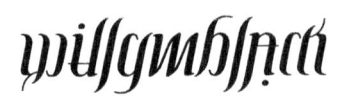

© Willy M Black · 2024 · All Rights Reserved
Cover design: **Pedro Delgado** · estornudo.es

DOES IT HURT WHEN I PRESS HERE TWO?

An A&E doctor's treatment for the NHS

WILLY M BLACK

INTRO

It is with great concern that I start writing the second part of this series. For several reasons. It seems like only those who have had a potentially life-changing medical condition or injury realise what an amazing thing it is to have a National Health Service (NHS). A service that will spare no resources in diagnosing and treating them, regardless of the cost and regardless of how little or how much that person has contributed to it through taxation or otherwise. "We don't appreciate what we've got" is a sentence these patients use when talking about their experience. Like everything in life, whether it's a partner, a friend, running water, a property or whatever, when something is there unconditionally, we tend to take it for granted, not really appreciating how fortunate we are. But as the Cinderella (the rock band, not the Disney character) song goes "Don't know what you got till it's gone." So please, do not wait until it's gone to treasure it, because when it's gone, it will be gone forever. Dentists, probably fed up with the abuse they receive and that they most definitely do not need to put up with to have a succulent income, are starting to withdraw their contracts with the NHS. When all dentists only see private paying patients, it will give those who did not appreciate what they had a good taste of what the NHS will eventually become if we let it happen. It will most definitely be a shame for those responsible users, but as usual, the selfish idiots fuck it all up for the rest of us.

Things have not only not got any better, but rather they have become much worse than in pre-pandemic times. In those times we were villains that became heroes. Now that most people feel safe again and we are not needed as much, we seem to have become supervillains of the worst kind.

The fact that General Practitioners (GPs) somehow managed to get away with hiding behind telephone consultations, avoiding patient contact in the times they were needed the most, probably is also to blame. Which other collective does that? Postal workers still delivered mail; bin men still collected our rubbish; supermarket staff served us every day without fail, whether selfish bastards had emptied the toilet roll shelves or not. Can you imagine soldiers refusing to fulfil their contract on what they are ultimately paid for, which is going to war? It is a nice thought, and I wish it would happen someday, but I hope you get my point. Needless to say, if there were delays in getting a GP appointment before the pandemic, now it is just an impossible quest. I would like to emphasize at this point that I am not familiar with the detailed dealings of a GP surgery and my opinion of what goes on in them is formed primarily from being at the receiving end of referrals and dissatisfied customers in the Emergency Department (ED). Let's not forget that we also get lots of people referred by the Surgery's receptionist, who has fuck all training in medicine or nursing so knows roughly as much about medicine as Bob the Builder. Working in close proximity with GPs does not magically give anyone medical knowledge, otherwise the cleaning staff would be as entitled to give medical advice. Considering that we are seeing an increasing number of attendees coming in, for example, for a routine wound dressing change after an operation, which historically has been done by Practice Nurses and is definitely not what an ED is for, please allow me to conclude that something has drastically changed in the way that GP surgeries operate. However, I would like to apologise in advance to GPs if I am being too harsh and invite them to start a healthy discussion on my Facebook page or Twitter account about any of the issues I refer to in this book. I might learn something I don't know, or even understand the hardships which I am sure they have to endure.

    I am also confident it has a lot to do with the deterioration of the mental health of the general population. This is what happens when the fear of death is constantly hyped up, drilled daily into the consciousness of the public, while depriving them of everything that humans need to keep sane, namely contact and interaction, hugs and kisses, socialising and laughter. Worth mentioning are attendances to the ED with functional disorders, whether they are pseudo-seizures, panic attacks, or any other presentation in which, although the person is convinced that there is something seriously wrong with them, there is no organic cause. We do take them seriously, we do investigate them, but invariably we find nothing of concern. That does not mean that there isn't a problem, it only means that there is not an emergency problem, therefore, we cannot be of any further help. It is like taking your car with an electrical problem to a tyre specialist: you can take it as many times as you like, but if there is nothing wrong with the tyres, they can't help. Patients take this as being dismissive or uncaring, and despite being pointed in the right direction, to get the right help, they keep coming over and over again, presenting with the same complaint. Instead of them seeking help from their GPs, the psychiatrists or mental health specialists, they keep returning to the ED, convinced that we are wrong or have missed something. By then we stop taking them seriously, how could we not? There is only so much you can sympathise with someone you have investigated over and over again with no abnormalities found. Ever. Which of course does not please them.

These two factors, the GP issue and the deterioration in mental health, when considered independently, are enough to increase the number of attendees to the ED, never mind when those same factors adversely influence each other, creating a loop of doom: then the damage can be considered in exponential terms. I have reiterated in my previous book that in the ED we are emergency physicians and not GPs, therefore we cannot refer patients for outpatient appointments or arrange investigations that are not urgent; we cannot treat conditions that are not accidents or life or limb threatening emergencies. And I really don't care if a person thinks that, for her, that abdominal pain that she has had for more than a year is an emergency that needs something doing at 3 in the morning on a Saturday. I think I should pay far less tax than I do, and yet the tax man does not give a fuck. And again, I am not saying that that person doesn't have a medical problem, I am just saying that we cannot help that person in the same way that an ophthalmologist (eye doctor) cannot help that same person with her stomach pain. And yes, I will say it again, we are all doctors, but for fuck's sake, people know that if they have a heart problem they need to see a cardiologist and not a gynaecologist, so why is the understanding of what an ED is any different? The ED is for emergencies and for emergencies only. Full stop. Believe me when I say that we really want to help you, our job is to help people and that is what makes us chose this profession. We will even go the extra mile and try to be of service to you in some way until you can get access to the professional or specialist that can either investigate your concerns appropriately or provide definitive treatment. To give you an example, we are not dentists, we know nothing about teeth, and if anyone has a dental problem, they should really see a dentist, the clue is in the name. But if for whatever reason they cannot and so attend the ED, we will not refuse to see them point blank: we will prescribe painkillers and antibiotics as a way of calming their pain and stopping the spread of infection until they can see a dentist that can sort them out. What other profession does that? If you consult a lawyer about something that is not within their area of expertise, they don't give you a little bit of legal advice until you find someone who can help you, they simply tell you to go and find advice somewhere else.

Another reason is the battered staff morale. A recent workforce survey by the Royal College of Emergency Medicine found that 50% of its members, that is half the doctors that run Emergency Departments, are considering reducing their working hours in the next two years, "largely due to workforce pressures and burnout." This is not only due to a lack of job satisfaction but also to the fact that, in the NHS, hard work is not appreciated, but rather the ability to keep quiet, be compliant with the ruling egos, look the other way, and not give a shit is. I have witnessed first-hand hitherto very motivated doctors and nurses who now have reached the end of their tether and cannot any longer give a fuck. Junior doctors that have studied hard to become doctors are now looking for alternative careers. On top of being already overworked, their load has massively increased while their salaries have not followed. A BBC News article dated 2nd April 2022 discusses how Milton Keynes Hospital has started a food exchange for staff struggling with the rising cost of living. "This is reality for many NHS staff," says Kate Jarman, Milton Keynes Hospital Corporate Affairs Director. They even had to call it *Food Exchange* so people would not feel embarrassed or uncomfortable using it. These are the same people that are there day and night, looking after anyone that needs medical care, sacrificing their social life, time with their families, their health both physical and mental, to be there for you. And don't get me wrong, I am not saying they do it just for those reasons, they are not nuns or charity workers. They have bills to pay and families to feed so they also do it for the money. But when a job is not worth its pay, people just leave. Think that a Health Care Assistant (HCA) gets paid per hour as much as a barista in Starbucks or a McDonalds worker. Yet they chose looking after people, with all the responsibilities and the crap (literally) that comes with it.

The fourth reason is the timing of the attendances. People coming to the ED at 2am with a pain they have had for 5 days, for no apparent logical reason, as in no worsening of the pain or no new symptoms. Conditions that are not emergencies, like an earache or a fever, can wait until the morning and should be dealt with by making a GP appointment. I know I have mentioned that seeing a GP is becoming an impossible quest, but that is no excuse to attend the ED. For years there have been Walk-In centres either attached to EDs or functioning on their own, and I have explained in my previous book what these centres are for. So here I propose another solution to the getting-an-appointment-with-your-GP problem which I believe would seem logical to anyone with more than 2 functioning neurons: GP surgeries could employ extra GPs and dedicate them solely to GP emergency appointments and home visits. As we are seeing, there is an increasing demand for GP appointments at any time of the day or night, so if we are to continue with the free-for-all current system, perhaps it is time to break away from the appointment system and extend this in-surgery emergency GP service to operate 24h, with an open-door policy like the ED or the out of hours GP services have, and no option to turn patients away without having first personally assessed them. Historically GPs have not operated out of hours because the conditions they deal with are not emergencies and can wait until the following day. The reality is that now these patients do not wait until the morning and instead, turn up in the ED, including nursing home residents who develop a fever or some minor condition. This approach would make much more sense than having people seen by random GPs, or in EDs where, and forgive me for repeating this so many times, we are not GPs, not to mention the number of resources or distress that would be saved to elderly folk with dementia by not being taken out of their familiar environment. I believe this to be a feasible plan of action, that would be inexpensive enough to be justified, and it would decongest the EDs in a massive way as well as providing access to patient's own GPs. I cannot be absolutely sure of why this has not been implemented, but my educated guess would be that there is no financial benefit for the surgery to do so, and since they are private enterprises that tend to prioritise whatever is profitable for them, whether it is reducing cholesterol levels in a percentage of their patients or getting them vaccinated, it would cost them money instead, and therefore, it would not be considered. This secondary problem would be sorted by the NHS taking over the management of GP surgeries and having salaried GPs working in them. So there you go.

    Complaints are supposed to be feedback systems with the aim of improving a service. I do tell patients to take the no-appointment issue up with their own GPs, to write to their Members of Parliament (MPs), to file complaints at their local surgery, even to write to the local newspaper. That might actually work, as opposed to attending the ED, which does not sort out anything, since their GPs get no feedback and therefore get the impression that they are providing a good service, and patients do not receive the help they need since attending the ED does not give them access to the right treatment. To my surprise, some even tell us that they attend in the early hours of the night thinking they are doing us a favour, as they thought it would be less busy at this time, but that just shows how little understanding the general public has of what an ED is for. I have already discussed this in my previous book, but I feel compelled to reiterate it, yet again: the ED is staffed 24h a day, every day of the year, including the extra days in leap years. This, however, does not mean that it is staffed equally after hours and during the night. Staffing levels, considering absences due to illness and posts not filled, is optimal, or close to, during working hours. From 22h to 8h, it functions at a basic level, to ensure that anyone with a life or limb threatening emergency gets medical care. This is a concept that should be self-explanatory. It is not operating 24/7 to make it easier for anyone to see a doctor whenever they see fit. Anyone attending the department at 3am with a sore throat, whether they think they are doing the ED a favour or not, is just putting unnecessary stress on the department and taking staff away from seeing to other patients that really need our attention.

Another cause for concern, the fifth one by my own count, is the seemingly ganging up of patients against members of staff, as if they knew better. This became worryingly apparent during the final months of the pandemic, when people were now not scared enough to not attend hospitals, like they were at the beginning, but the access restrictions, meaning no relatives allowed into the department, were still in place. Of course, there were exceptions, like disabled patients or even those who could not speak English; this latter one was hugely abused by non-British born citizens pretending not to understand English for it later to become clear that they could both understand and speak it fluently when denied entry with a companion, but hey, just another example of the extent of the abuse. Whether we agree with these restrictions or not is irrelevant. If we don't follow the rules imposed on us by management, we get the bollocking, not them, they always get the apology letter. So we have no choice and there is nothing positive to gain by arguing with us. Those in the waiting room (WR) who had witnessed a relative come in as one of the exceptional cases I have mentioned, now start arguing, trying to get their companions in with them, raising their voices as if they were fighting the good fight. We had people furiously shouting at us that they did not agree with those rules. As if we gave a fuck what rules they agree with or not. Do these same people see a red traffic light and think "fuck that, I don't agree with the highway code" and drive through it? Do they shout at the police when caught, stopped and fined? Or do they get a letter from HMRC informing them that they owe money in tax and go "fuck that, I don't agree with your tax rules" and then not pay? Do they get an appointment to see their GP and turn up whenever they want because they don't agree with the time slot? Perhaps they refuse to go through security at the airport, however ridiculous the rules are regarding the amount of liquids or the size of the see-through plastic bag? I very much doubt it. They seem to only feel entitled in the ED and I suspect it has a lot to do with the fact that they have been allowed to feel and act that way.

The NHS receives far more complaints than any other public institution, and every complaint is taken seriously, even if unjustified or a plain lie. I have never heard of patients apologising, or being made to apologise under warning of being banned from a hospital for making unjustified complaints, being rude or even assaulting a member of staff, but I have heard of Trusts forcing employees to call patients to apologise for, for example, not requesting an x-ray that was not indicated in the first place, or telling them that what they are presenting with is not an emergency, often with the aim of pointing them in the right direction but usually taken as offence. When you speed on the motorway, you get a fine, kind of telling you that you must not drive over the speed limit, so you don't do it again. You can complain as much as you want and still won't get an apology, and you better pay that fine in time. You can call the fire brigade to complain about a noisy neighbour and you probably will be politely told to fuck off. Again, you can complain as much as you want, but you will receive no apology. The most absurd I have heard is a complaint made by a patient who took offense after a member of staff sprayed some air freshener in an area that was thick with the smell of faeces, stale body odour and a diabetic ulcer. I am unclear of whether the smells were all coming from the same patient and which of the patients complained.

I have experienced this ganging up attitude myself when I have called patients in from the WR attending with, say, a thumb injury, or a headache, by ambulance, of course, and put by the kind paramedics in a wheelchair. There is absolutely no reason why that person should be in a wheelchair, and this is a topic that I also dedicated a whole chapter to in my previous book. The fact that a person is in a hospital does not mean that they surrender all autonomy to us: they can still walk, talk, insert their suppositories into their own rectums and wipe their own arses afterwards. But just because they have been sat in a wheelchair, they expect to be wheeled around and, well, I refuse to play that game. Therefore, I patiently wait for them to get up and walk, like in a pigeon fight: we stare at each other to see who gives in first. In the meantime, all the do-gooders in the WR start moving their heads in indignation, commenting some bollocks about the quality of the service, and even pushing the chair towards me and giving me the look. "This person cannot walk" they tell me, because the person is in a wheelchair, can you not see that doctor? All those years of medical school didn't do much good, did they? Of course, I cannot tell them what the presenting problem is, that is confidential, and I want to think that if I could reveal the nature of it, even the do-gooders would think the person in the wheelchair is a cunt, taking a chair unnecessarily that could be used by Mrs Woodcock, 83, attending with massively swollen legs. It really beats me why anyone would think that we do this on purpose, with the malicious intent to cause further harm or discomfort to a patient, but I guess it is no different than thinking that we do not order a CT scan or an x-ray or a blood test, not because it is not indicated, but because we are evil fuckers, daredevils that take pleasure in jeopardising our jobs. As an added piece of information, we don't pay for the scans, or any tests we order for that matter, from our own pockets and we really don't give a rat's arse how much money is spent on a patient, but there is this thing called the *Ionising Radiation (Medical Exposure) Regulations 2017* that makes us accountable for any radiation we expose our patients to. I don't think anyone goes to a restaurant with the first impression that the waiter is going to give them shit service or that the chef is going to prepare them an awfully bad tasting meal. I don't believe for a minute that people would take their car to the garage expecting to have more faults once it has been serviced. So why are we so different when it comes to people's expectations of us?

In any case, I make the patient get up and follow me. Invariably, after all the drama created, they get up and act as if they were dizzy, which makes no fucking sense, I have read their triage notes and no dizziness is mentioned as the cause for their injury, although it is a good performance for those knobs who are indignantly still shaking their heads. This dizziness and holding-on-to-things bullshit suddenly resolves as they enter the department and are out of sight of the kind-hearted Samaritans in the WR. They then magically walk in a straight line and all. After sorting them out, having forgotten about their "dizziness", I walk out with them, their gait instability having miraculously resolved. My intention is to prove a point to all those head-nodding idiots that think they are kind and caring persons, although they probably still think that the dizziness was real, and it's now resolved because I have treated the patient for that. But can you understand our predicaments? And that is only something as simple as calling someone in to be seen. Imagine the conflict generated when they want a test that is not indicated, and we tell them so. Whatever we do, it's a losing battle.

So please do help us, and by helping us you will be helping yourself. You are just a passive witness of what is going on. We are professionals in health. We have information that you don't have. We have skills that you lack. You can see someone, for instance, having a fit in the WR and think it is outrageous that no one is really doing anything about it. If that is the case, be reassured that if that person was having a proper generalised tonic-clonic seizure we would be there in a flash. If no one is doing anything about it, it's because we know this patient, or have triage information already, and those seizures you see are not real, and therefore do not require any emergency assistance. What we are doing is making sure that that person is not jumping the queue and that everyone is being seen and treated according to priority and waiting times. Having an argument with us about it doesn't help anyone and even makes things worse, because that person is learning a behaviour that ends up in personal reward and it is also unnecessarily prolonging the time that others have to wait to be seen, not to mention upsetting members of staff that probably still have many hours left of their shift. We are not tin men, we do have hearts and feelings, and no one works at their 100% when upset. Please understand that we are health professionals because we care, not because we find pleasure in neglecting our patients. But people know this already, otherwise they wouldn't come to see us. Allow us to do our job. Amongst the apparent chaos there is an order that makes sense to us.

One more reason I can think of, the sixth and final for now, is the aftereffects of the disastrous management of the Sars-Cov-2 pandemic, with its lockdowns and school closures, with the lack of human interaction and the consequent adverse effects on our immune systems. It is neither a new nor a revolutionary concept that the best immunity is acquired by being exposed to bacteria and viruses. Same applies with the need for continuous training and testing of our immune cells, which like athletes, need frequent re-exposures to maintain a decent level of expertise. That is the history of us and our surroundings. The Bubonic Plague of 1346, also known as the Black Death, subsided because the people that were exposed to it and survived developed immunity to the causing pathogen, the bacteria Yersinia pestis, little by little during the 7 years that the pandemic lasted, in a time where hygiene was non-existent, until their immune systems learnt how to keep it at bay. Malaria, in endemic countries, does not affect the locals in the same way that it affects visitors that have never been exposed to the malaria parasite. However, if a local moves to a non-malaria country, their immune system slowly "forgets" how to fight the Plasmodium, and if infected on returning after several years abroad, the infection will be far more severe. This, no more and no less, is what we are seeing at the time of writing with the yearly influenza, with common colds that seem to now affect us more intensely, and definitely with the way Strep A/Scarlet Fever started affecting children in an unprecedented way. No rocket science, but basic medical knowledge, ignored by those who know fuck all about medicine or immunology or virology for the sake of being seen to be doing something. Praising the Sars-Cov-2 vaccines for helping to end the pandemic situation without a properly conducted study that includes a control group, namely the unvaccinated, is completely misleading. If we use that unscientific approach, any intervention that precedes an improvement in any illness, whether it is homeopathy, reiki, shaking bones, or giving antibiotics to combat a viral infection, has to be praised for such improvement. We only have to look at countries, specifically African countries, where the vaccination uptake has not been above 5% of the population and yet, Sars-Cov-2 does not seem to have affected them that much worse than it affected us.

I hear voices saying that the solution to the NHS crisis is privatisation, or at least introducing charges for the services. Myself and everyone I work with as far as I know, have always been against any sort of privatisation of the NHS because ultimately the ones that will suffer the most will be precisely those who use the service appropriately. The time wasters will stop coming and they won't suffer since their conditions are not real emergency conditions at all, but those who only attend the ED when they genuinely need medical attention will be penalised and I will never agree with a system that does that. Having said that, a system that allows a perfectly healthy child to be brought to the ED by their worried parents 10 times before their first birthday, or a healthy adult to seek medical attention several times a month is a non-viable system that is doomed to collapse.

Sadly, the awful reality is that opinions are changing among healthcare staff. Those of us that care are there fighting for the NHS to improve, but we are also there in the front line taking all the abuse and all the crap from every front. So, sadly, as I said, the winds are changing and "I can't wait for the NHS to be privatised" is a statement that is heard increasingly coming from those who are exhausted from a fight in which those that we are defending are also against us. It really feels like doing the impossible for the ungrateful. So what is the fucking point? Privatisation might come in the way that is practised in the US, which makes us cringe in the UK, or, I believe, a much fairer system would be to implement a fixed fee, let's say £50 to start with, per attendance, regardless of employment or disability status. That, I am sure, would make people think twice, perhaps take some painkillers and see if that sorts out the pain and stop using the "I am sure it is nothing but I just wanted to get it checked" card.

Before we jump onto the next chapter, I would like to leave you with a thought. I have mentioned the reasons why I think ED departments all around the country are getting busier with attenders with non-emergency complaints. I have listed the reasons that are contributing to this, but if we make a comparison with pre-pandemic times, we saw a huge decrease in attendances when we didn't know what kind of illness COVID-19 was. It was lovely in the ED, because we were just seeing emergencies, which is what we really really like and what the department is for. The regular attenders decreased the frequency of their visits; even the regular overdosers, in such unprecedented times of fear and uncertainty, somehow stopped taking tablets galore. No one came with minor complaints. People still had the same headaches, the same belly pains, the sore throats and earaches that overwhelmed the EDs before the pandemic. They still fell and had cuts and bruises, but they treated them at home. They probably took greater care when de-stoning avocados. Somehow the fear of an unknown illness gave people common sense. Or maybe it was just that it made them scared of hospitals. As our knowledge of the virus and the disease progressed, the attendances started to increase, including overdosers, regular attenders and the rest. That alone, speaks for itself.

PROLOGUE

The other day, while listening to a patient's chest, I couldn't help but feel amazed by how wonderful it is to have a National Health Service. The patient in question was dressed in very ragged clothes. He was 76, had no past medical history and took no medication. A hard-working farmer, who still enjoyed working on his farm, that had a sudden onset of chest pain and got a bit concerned. He hadn't used the service much, his GP probably didn't even know him, but he knew that should he need medical assistance, he would have limitless access and care. When we compare our NHS with the systems in place in countries like the United States of America, the greatest country in the world (although that's according to them), where diabetics have to ration their insulin, even die because they can't afford their life saving treatment, or Venezuela, where people with gunshot wounds are taken to a hospital and left to die unless they can prove they have medical insurance, we should be ashamed of allowing our National Health Service to become what it has become: a system where an ambulance is called by members of the public to avoid paying for a taxi, or by primary care professionals in panic; where patients, even the unemployed on benefits, shout at staff that they pay their salary (are politicians reminded of this too?); where any amount of good is suddenly erased into oblivion by an expectation not met; where the workers are punished by everyone, including those they are fighting for; where rewarding experiences are overwhelmingly outnumbered by frustrating ones.

An Emergency Department should be full of people with broken bones and legs in Plaster of Paris, having cardiac arrests and heart attacks, fitting, bleeding from wounds requiring a lot of pressure, even tourniquets, to control the haemorrhage, looking pale, vomiting profusely, their skin covered in cold sweat. ED staff should be jumping from one patient to the next, recording their vital signs, listening to their chests, palpating their abdomens, administering intravenous analgesia, fluids, antibiotics, with someone passionately shouting in the background "Adrenaline, 1mg, STAT" or "Put more pressure on that bleed!"

Instead, today's ED is full of people that have registered with complaints such as *cough and fever for a few days*, or *abdominal pain for 3 months*, or *gastroenteritis*, or *chicken pox*, or with imaginary illnesses in which they faint, or have numbness all over the body, or cannot move their legs for no apparent reason. Complaints that make no sense to an experienced clinician, for they seem to disappear when nobody is paying attention; pains that move following impossible pathways, and symptoms that do not fit into any known syndrome, as if any minor deviation from normal health, whether objective or self-perceived, were a reason to call for an ambulance and seek medical assistance. Patients lie on trolleys reading books, looking either like dying ducks or absolutely not ill at all, happily playing on their mobile phones while casually drinking cups of tea, talking to their relatives on loudspeaker annoying everyone around them with their conversation, or watching movies, a few even in their comfy pyjamas, as if they were lying on their living room sofa. Some of them come to the nurses' station every now and then to let us know how concerned they are about another patient not having been taken to the toilet or to point out that the telephone has been ringing repeatedly and none of the nurses have stopped administering treatments, moving patients to wards or checking whether they have pressure sores to answer it. Paramedics walk in, smiling, holding in their arms a little child with a face in awe as if they had just arrived in Disneyland, or bring in a bloke laughing and making jokes strapped to an ambulance trolley. Someone is shouting "please help me!" about 10,000 times per minute, usually an elderly person, extremely frightened, who has been taken out of their familiar environment and sent to the ED with some bullshit condition because the nursing home they reside in is short staffed tonight, or the GP on the phone thought that it would be better for the patient to be transported by ambulance rather than him/her actually visiting the patient and saving resources and distress. Speaking of resources,

3 members of staff, including security, are busy dealing with Kevin, a regular attender who, after getting pissed out of his head, like he does every other day, started shouting in the middle of the street that he was going to kill himself, resulting in the usual call to 999 by bystanders and the subsequent trip to the ED, only to now make a fuss because he wants to leave and is going to sue everybody. Samantha, a 32-year-old frequent flyer has "fainted" and conveniently placed herself in the middle of the corridor's floor obstructing the flow of trolleys and point-blank refuses to move. She has drunk a bottle of vodka this morning and phoned the police letting them know that she was going to kill herself, only to then abscond, leaving the police with the burden and responsibility of urgently searching for her. When tired of not being found, she entered a restaurant and took a fistful of pills in front of everyone, resulting, as it happens, in an ambulance being called, and here she is, getting shit loads of attention and making everybody's job more difficult than it already is. In reception, a mother who has registered her child with "nappy rash for 3 weeks" is complaining that they have been waiting for 3 hours to see a doctor, although she only registered 62 minutes ago. When told that patients are seen according to priority, she says that her baby, of course, is a priority. She threatens with making a complaint and is asking the receptionist for her name. A woman in her 30s is demanding that the hospital pays for her taxi home since she "didn't want to come but the ambulance brought her here", while a male in his mid-50s that did want to come by ambulance with a history of abdominal pain for 3 months that he hasn't thought much of but now is worried about, is shouting that he will discharge himself if he is not seen immediately. During all this, doctors and nurses continue with their carrot-on-a-stick quest to reduce the waiting times and hopefully, clear the department. It is 3:25 in the morning and half of the nurses on the night shift haven't even had time to have a toilet break.

To support what you have just read, I would love to take photos at work and illustrate this book with pictures of people with neck collars sat on their trolleys facetiming a mate or taking pictures of themselves having intravenous fluids to post on social media, but that would get me in a lot of trouble. So next time you are unfortunate enough to require medical attention in an ED, just take the time to look around and check it out for yourself. It is quite amusing to witness what the ED has become. And it can only get worse because we keep lowering the line of the presentations we will attend to. We shouldn't be seeing people that come to the ED after an injury without bothering to take painkillers first; we shouldn't be removing contact lenses that are not misplaced or broken from people's eyes; we should not be dressing wounds that could be done at home; we shouldn't be removing splinters or ticks from people, there are loads of videos online explaining how to remove them with simple measures that anyone can do. And yet, we are expected to do all of these. Are we going to start scratching people's backs when they cannot reach the itchy spot? Are we going to change nappies for babies when parents claim they don't know how to change them? Perhaps offer appointments to give them their feeds? If the NHS was a National Electricity Service, people would call an electrician out to change a bulb.

People used to understand that if they suffered from a chronic illness, having bouts every now and then was part of it. Like being epileptic and having a fit every now and then; or suffering from angina and having an attack that resolves by resting or taking a couple of puffs of GTN under the tongue. In the world of today, epileptics have a simple uncomplicated fit or angina patients have a short-lived attack and end up in the ED. They usually come by ambulance, I suspect courtesy of 111, they wait to be seen, and they are sent home as they came, since we cannot treat what is normal for a patient in the context of a chronic condition. The NHS was designed when there was a common sense amongst the population that dictated that if anyone had gastroenteritis, it would involve diarrhoea, vomiting, abdominal pain, and general malaise for a few days; if suffering from a seasonal flu, then back, limbs and head were going to hurt, there will be coughing and the person will feel awful. And all anyone can do about it is to have some rest and take some home remedies, chicken soup, or over-the-counter medication to ease the symptoms. If a child had chicken pox, or cried all night, mothers knew what to do, and tried everything to calm the baby. In today's world, people suffering from these ailments come to the ED as if they were going to Lourdes or Fatima, expecting a miracle that would make it all pass in the blink of an eye. It truly feels like people cannot have a fall or a minor cut, sprain their ankle or wrist, or even have a tiny splinter, without seeking medical attention. You might remember the case I mentioned in my previous book about a patient attending the ED to have her contact lenses removed, which by the way, more colleagues have since professed to "treating" similar cases, fake nails being so popular. Today's children cannot have childhood viral illnesses, or cry all night, without the worried parents taking them to be checked by an ED doctor in the middle of the night, in a *just in case* fashion. Not to mention all the potential damage that can be done to pregnant ladies, or rather their unborn babies, and immunocompromised patients, by taking a child to a hospital with an infective viral illness like chicken pox, as well as all the stuff babies can catch from other patients. The system is not designed to cope with every little injury or every worsening of every chronic disease, hence the overwhelmingly broken and rotten state it is in now. At this pace, it won't be long before every migraine or irritable bowel sufferer comes to the ED with every headache or episode of belly pain. The same applies to minor abrasions and contusions, as it feels like people cannot have any minor injury anymore and just treat it at home. Our grandmothers would be ashamed.

ED departments can be sustainable only if they do what they are designed to do, which is dealing with accidents, trauma and life or limb threatening emergencies. Can you imagine a delivery ward full of people with non-maternity related illnesses? First, the doctors would not be skilled in dealing with those illnesses and the pregnant women about to have their babies would not be looked after as they should be. Why is the ED treated so differently to every other specialist service?

One of the biggest problems we face, as practitioners, is that medicine is not an exact science, like physics or mathematics are. There is no always, there is no never and 2 plus 2 does not always equal 4. We work on probabilities, always balancing risks against benefits in everything we do. It is in the "there is no never" where the problem lies, as it means that anything can be possible. Even what only happens to 1 in a billion people happens to 1 person out of a billion people. Having said that, it is not possible to investigate every patient for every rare condition that we know of. Take cancer screening for example: although breast cancer can affect people of all ages, including men, screening in the UK is only offered to women between the ages of 50 and 71. Every age group has its extensively documented conditions that we focus on when we are in the process of diagnosing. This is what we consider normal, like for instance, having heart attacks, strokes or dementia after 70. Different types of tachyarrhythmias (rapid heartbeats, regular or irregular) have their target age groups too, with first presentations of atrial fibrillation being to the elderly what first presentations of Wolf-Parkinson-White are to children or adolescents. Hip pains in children around 4 to 10 years of age make us think of Perthe's disease, while the same symptoms in slightly older teens make us think of slipped capital femoral epiphysis (SCFE). Healthy children and young adults don't suffer from dementia, or have heart attacks, but we can never say it is an absolute impossibility. However, proceeding to investigate any condition that falls outside what we consider normal without a justifiable level of concern would be an inappropriate use of resources that a) the system is not equipped to deal with and b) would result in unnecessary radiation and unnecessary exposure to other risks. Imagine hospital beds being taken by children with chest pain being investigated for heart attacks, having invasive procedures that carry a 1 in a 1000 risk of death and being given medications in the meantime that affect their blood pressure and the way their blood clots; or by adults that have had a cough for 2 days and so are going through the process of having their chest looked at by either scans that expose them to a huge amount of radiation or cameras down their windpipes when the likelihood of a heart attack in a child and lung cancer in someone that has coughed for 2 days are as close to zero as it gets. I invite anyone who still does not understand what I've just explained to honestly think if they would go ahead and ask for these investigations if they had to pay for them from their own pocket. I could carry on with lots of other examples, but I hope that you can understand the point I am trying to make.

If we add to this any degree of malingering, hypochondria or even imaginary illnesses, now labelled functional disorders, in mental health patients, then things can get really confusing. There is a new concept, cyberchondria, where people look up conditions online and apply what's called *confirmation bias* to reinforce the suspicion that there is something serious going on. For example, a person suffering from a headache and sicky feeling can do a quick search on the NHS website for Brain Tumours. The search will produce a list of common symptoms such as headaches, seizures (fits), persistently feeling sick (nausea), being sick (vomiting), drowsiness, mental or behavioural changes such as memory problems or changes in personality, progressive weakness or paralysis on one side of the body and vision or speech problems. They will then take their 2 symptoms out of the 8 and, through the forementioned process of *confirmation bias* ignore the other 6 rather important symptoms and self-diagnose with a brain tumour with a consequent visit to the ED.

Anyone can call an ambulance, say that they have suddenly lost their vision, or that they cannot move, or talk, and there is always a rare presentation of some illness that can produce that particular symptom. Of course, it has to be in context, as in part of a syndrome or associated with other signs, which a good clinician will recognise and will not be misled. But ED staff, through complaints and fear of investigation by a regulatory body, namely the General Medical Council (GMC) or the Royal College of Nursing (RCN) have been conditioned to avoid taking the responsibility of using their knowledge or thinking outside the box (more on this later) and to actually believe or treat any presentation as genuine. Malingerers know of this systemic weakness and how to exploit it. They can threaten to throw themselves in front of a bus if not given a free ride home and be granted that free ride. They can pretend that they can't move their legs to get a bed in hospital, or faint to jump the queue and be seen quicker. The fainting itself, or any of the other symptoms mentioned, will make no sense in the context of whatever it is that the patient is complaining of, so it will mislead the doctor in trying to reach a diagnosis. This will inevitably result in extra time spent with that particular patient and inappropriate use of resources and investigations, which might confuse the picture even further. The NHS itself does not reward members of staff that treat malingerers as malingerers, it punishes them perhaps in an attempt to clear the Trust's responsibility and rather blame a rogue individual. Ambulances have been used as taxis for those living near a hospital area for their return journey after a night out. I have heard of people visiting cities and rather than paying for a hotel, attending the local ED with some bullshit, sleeping over to self-discharge in the morning and continue with their business. It begs the question of why homeless people sleep rough when they could make use of this loophole. The truth is that all they would have to do is claim to have any of these mentioned symptoms to be able to sleep, at least, in the ED. This is how your taxes are spent, how the money that should be used to provide quality medical care ends, in a considerable proportion, spent on malingerers, selfish motherfuckers that could not care less whether a 90-year-old nan has to sleep in a chair because they have taken the last available bed with their bullshit illness. Anyone who attempts to sort this situation out, who wants to use the resources appropriately, who is efficient, is seen as a nuisance that makes others look lazy and therefore is punished, deemed a daredevil, and quickly conditioned to adapt to the existing patterns and to not give a shit. Because in the NHS if you give a shit, the person you report to does not, which makes you a disturbance, a white noise in an otherwise nice managerial job. "Please stop telling me how the service that you provide could be improved, made more efficient and fairer for all users. My life is difficult enough as it is, and I don't want any headaches. I know you are encouraged to report any safety issues and all that crap, but please fuck off and report them to someone else." You might remember the same modus operandi described in my previous book when it comes to whistle-blowers, so this should be no surprise.

As you can see, our voices are not being heard, our safety concerns lost in a sea of apathy, so you should be angry, very angry. In fact, you should be furious and it should encourage you to take action. Considering that people make complaints for pretty much any fucking thing, for instance, about members of staff looking at them funny, or for being told they shouldn't be there, or most of the time not even for being told, but for being made to feel as if they shouldn't be in the department (I am sorry, but if a condition is not an emergency, we cannot treat it as an emergency), no one, however, seems to be bothered or make any complaints about the Hospital or the Trust not being firm on dangerous attenders or time wasters, who at the end of the day, are responsible for, or at least contribute to, the long wait that you, with a genuine complaint, have to endure. You pay taxes to receive a decent service, and that's what you should get, so I urge you, if you witness any incidents of this sort, any problematic attenders abusing members of staff, or making you feel uncomfortable, to write a complaint to the Hospital, demanding that incidents like that are taken seriously. No one cares about us, no one gives a shit if we are assaulted, threatened or humiliated at work, but your voice is always heard, your concerns always addressed, you always get the apology letter. Consider that incidents of this type are regular occurrences, and I guarantee you that if you asked how many people the Hospital have banned in the last few years, or even in the last decade, for being disrespectful, abusive, or for making other patients feel in danger, the response will be zero. Nil. None. Ninguno.

Sorry, I got carried away with the malingerers and time wasters, but it had to be said. Now, back to the issue of medicine not being an exact science, you might argue that precisely what I have explained is reason enough for people to seek medical attention after a simple sneeze, but then you might as well bring your slippers and move into the hospital. Our bodies tell us when we need water, or food, or a dump, or to empty our bladders. Our bodies tell us when rest or sleep is needed, or when we need to come back to the surface and refill our lungs after a dive. People don't go and lie in bed just in case they need to sleep. In the same way, our bodies tell us when something is really wrong. Anything else, for instance, a painful tooth, a mole that now has started to itch or bleed, being hungrier and thirstier than normal all the time, or passing blood when peeing, requires the same level of self-responsibility as, for example, men examining their own testicles regularly feeling for lumps. If it is an emergency, you will know, and if it is not normal, since you know what is normal for you, you will also know. I would like to take this opportunity to please ask that if you are a man, do not attend the ED asking for a "just in case" examination of your balls. That is something you can do yourself, it is fun, and who knows what it might lead to. Wink wink. If you are a woman, please follow the usual recommendations to get your boobs checked and your smear tests regularly.

Us doctors cannot base our practice on the exceptions, like you cannot stop going out because someone got killed once from being hit by a small meteorite, or because around 400 pedestrians are killed by cars every year in the UK. Consider that, rarely, planes fall on houses, so staying at home does not guarantee your safety either. No system can cope with a great number of people wanting to get checked *just in case*. A good way of deciding whether to attend the ED would be to imagine whether you would still go if you had to pay the £160 that every attendance costs the taxpayer from your own pocket, even if that is the advice of the 111 operator. Apply the same rule when being taken to hospital by ambulance: the cost is £255 just for the ambulance, then add the £160 for the ED attendance. You came by ambulance and are discharged with only advice; it will be £415 sir. Would you like to pay cash or card?

It is starting to feel like the ED is that place where some people go to feel important and get the attention that they lack in their everyday life. Like when it is a special occasion and dinner in a nice restaurant is booked maybe involving flowers, or a box of chocolates, or a day at the spa. In the ED it's like that: everybody by default will treat patient's kindly and with respect, no matter how much abuse they throw at staff, how much noise they make, how much they complain or how much of a cunt that person is. These people own the place and act accordingly. That is why they feel entitled to tell us, even command us, how to run the department. That is why that patient that was concerned about another patient not having been taken to the toilet feels it is his duty to express his concerns. It makes me wonder whether when in a restaurant he also tells the waiter that the table next door has been waiting for their food for half an hour, or whether he feeds every homeless person he encounters. I suspect not. People tend to be more prone to throwing abuse at others when they know that those others cannot talk back.

The NHS and particularly the ED is that place where giving a hand inevitably ends in losing the whole arm, the whole body and even the dignity of those who work hard to be there for those same people that take it all. More frequently shouts of demands end in "now!" as if the demander didn't only own the place and the system, but also those that are employed by it. If you ask me, the solution to this abusive, even illegal treatment of NHS workers is 2 tier: first, and allow me to reiterate that you need to get involved in this too, people (patients and staff) need to have the balls to demand that it stops, that enough is enough. But instead, staff put up with it and patients don't seem to care. Second, the people that can do something about it work in offices in a galaxy far far away from the ED, seldom pay visits to the department, and are usually under the impression that we are not doing our job. They would love to have a slave trader with a whip, lashing at the nurses and doctors to work harder, faster, with no breaks, later blaming them for the mistakes they've made out of tiredness and putting them through hell after a dissatisfied customer complains. On paper it is all about quality care, but in reality it's about sausage-factory conveyer-belt style. Heisenberg's principle dictates that you have to choose between knowing the speed or the location of an electron, that you cannot accurately determine both. In the same way, you cannot have quality care, excellent medical treatment, while having it conveniently fast. One of the two have to give, to compromise, to make way for the other. Paradoxically, patients don't seem to understand this principle, and demand the impossibility of having both, so they also don't seem to give a shit. Patients keep coming with minor ailments even when junior doctors are on strike and the rest of us have to keep the boat afloat. So, there you go, balls and giving a shit. That is the simple and only solution. So please, help us out on this.

To put things into perspective, you can call a private dentist to book an appointment to be seen for a dental abscess, and they can choose not to see you. If you develop any complications from it and suffer harm, even death, the dentist will have no responsibility whatsoever. This applies to GPs too, and for that matter, to the ophthalmologists in the Eye Clinic if you presented with a problem not related to the eye. They can always play the *Go to A&E* card. This same principle does not apply to the ED: everyone attending the ED is seen, regardless of whether their complaint is a life or limb threatening emergency or not a medical complaint at all. If someone went to the ED and registered saying that they have just opened their bowels and need someone to wipe their arse, they will have their arse wiped.

As a rule, in a system that is not looked after by anyone, not even by its users and, as a consequence of this permanent neglect, is understaffed and therefore busy beyond capacity, the service that the users receive is bound to be suboptimal, whether that means not receiving analgesia on time, not having a trolley to be examined on, preserving some degree of dignity, long waits, or even having a blood test or an x-ray that is not really needed. It is getting to a point where suboptimal would actually be desirable. I mentioned in my previous book the reasons why it is both permanently understaffed and busy beyond capacity, and considering that this is the opposite of what it needs to be when its purpose is to deal with patient's health and lives and deliver quality care, as is always the aim, very little is being done to improve the situation. Probably because the people that make decisions at the highest levels, namely politicians, have access to private health care and are not really that bothered about the health problems of us, the plebs, regardless of their promises when voting time is around the corner.

At the time of writing, newspaper front covers are filled with headlines of long waiting times and queues of ambulances waiting patiently to offload their patients. I can guarantee you that more than half of those patients waiting to be offloaded did not need any treatment en-route to the hospital and could have made their own way either by themselves or at least as a passenger in a car or taxi, rather than taking up an ambulance unnecessarily. My proposed solution would be for paramedics to refuse to take to the ED anyone that should be checked by a doctor but is fit to make their own way in a car and does not require any treatment en-route. That alone, would stop a great number of inappropriate attendances. I am not claiming any credit for this solution as it is neither an original nor a novel idea: it is practiced in pretty much every European country I know of.

An ED is designed so that any serious emergency can be guaranteed medical attention always, but there is this fucked up notion that the ED is operative 24h a day every day of the year so people can have access to a doctor for any minor ailment any time they want. I am aware that the great majority of people do seek medical advice and use the resources appropriately, but unfortunately most of the people we see in the ED are those that attend at any time, day or night, for anything. So in my line of work it is hard not to be biased and believe that everybody is a time waster. Calling an ambulance for any minor fucking thing and, surprisingly enough, being transported to hospital for that same minor complaint, has become so the norm that my heart melts every time a patient with an asthma attack or serious chest pain makes their own way to the department because they didn't think their condition "was serious enough to request an ambulance". They didn't want to use resources that they understand are for prehospital care when other patients have conditions that require immediate treatment. In the same way, my blood boils when someone with a hangover calls an ambulance because they "feel weird". I did discuss this subject in depth in my previous book, so I am not going to bore you with the details again. Also, just writing about it is making my blood pressure go up. There is also the issue of everything being free. Let me explain: we can rule out, let's say, a fractured ankle by clinical examination. But people don't seem to trust our clinical skills, so they demand an x-ray. When they see that we are deciding that an x-ray is not needed, pains appear where before there was none. An ankle x-ray, 2 views, costs an average of £110 at private clinics in the UK. If people demanding x-rays had to pay for them, they would kiss the doctor that deems them unnecessary on clinical grounds. But because they can get it for free, they demand it is done.

Anyway, the point that I was trying to make is that, in this line of work, it is easy to mistakenly convince yourself that the attendees represent the whole of the population, like it is easy to believe that de-stoning an avocado is the most dangerous kitchen activity ever and that every motorcyclist dies on the road. So please forgive me if I sound more bitter than in my previous book. I once heard from a junior doctor the paradox of how working in the ED to help people turns into a dislike for people that had never been experienced before. So to make up for this, I would like to dedicate this book to you, for using the healthcare system responsibly, for doing your very best to stop it from collapsing and for helping reduce the number of alcoholics and suicide victims among NHS staff. Please do not feel offended by my statements and my swearing. It is not directed at you. You are the kind of good person the world needs more of. Cheers.

In my previous book, the aim was to diagnose the NHS; in this second part, I aim to propose treatments and solutions that will both work and make the system sustainable and viable for what it was originally designed to do.

Now, the disclaimer about this being a work of fiction and any resemblance with reality is purely coincidental, as stated in my previous book, still applies. The patients' stories told in this book, all of them true, although written in the first person, are often stories experienced by other doctors, but made my own for the purpose of making the narrative easier to follow. If you have not read my first book, feel free to go ahead and buy it. It is rather good, even if I do say so myself, and readers usually leave complementary reviews. If you have already read it, liked it and you also enjoy reading this one, feel free to recommend them to everyone you know (please do) and perhaps buy them as a present for someone you know will enjoy or will learn something from reading them. I am on X and Facebook and would love to hear from you. Also, the royalties and following would take me a step further in fulfilling my dream of becoming a full-time writer.

2. The primary duty of all doctors is for the care and safety of patients. Whatever their role, doctors must do the following […]

    b. Contribute to discussions and decisions about improving the quality of services and outcomes.
    c. Raise and act on concerns about patient safety. […]
    g. Use resources efficiently for the benefit of patients and the public. […]

16. Whether you have a management role or not, your primary duty is to patients. Their care, dignity and safety must be your first concern. […]

24. Early identification of problems or issues with the performance of individuals, teams or services is essential to help protect patients.

(Extract from the GMC's DUTIES OF A DOCTOR IN THE WORKPLACE)
https://www.gmc-uk.org/ethical-guidance/ethical-guidance-for-doctors/leadership-and-management-for-all-doctors/duties-of-a-doctor-in-the-workplace

Stepping into my shoes (Part 1)

It does not matter how many Emergency Department reality TV shows you watch, or whether you are a fan of Grey's Anatomy or follow any other TV series about my job: no one can really understand what it is to be a doctor unless you are one. No one can understand the level of responsibility that a doctor agrees to take on with every single patient.

In this chapter I would like to invite you into my shoes for a shift, in an attempt to convey what our day to day is like. I will spare you the worry that we take home with us about whether we have misdiagnosed or done everything possible for every one of our patients, the concerns about whether management is counting the number of patients that we saw during the shift or even how this affects our social life, our sleep and our mental health. The routines and cases that I will describe usually overlap. Sometimes a doctor is dealing with 3 to 5 patients at the same time, kind of like a waiter attending to several tables at once, moving from one to the other while tests are being processed, reviewing each one of the patient's progress and/or response to treatment, thinking of other differential diagnoses, writing notes and results, being pestered by management to make decisions quicker, being interrupted to sign ECGs for other patients, prescribe painkillers or iv fluids for someone we haven't even met, and being asked to urgently review a patient that one of the nurses is concerned about. And all whilst making sure that the customer that ordered the Tuna Salad doesn't get the Beef Wellington. I've written it all in a linear kind of way, describing only cases that were a bit more challenging to manage, to make it easier for you to remember who is who and what is what. So here we go.

On arriving in the department, the first thing we tend to do is look at the number of ambulances parked in the ambulance bay, and the amount of people in the waiting room. Most days, just looking at this is enough to ruin our shift. Invariably there will be at least one person in each of these categories: someone in handcuffs accompanied by a couple of police officers; someone laying on the floor with or without a bowl full of vomit by their side; someone that starts moaning in pain as they see us walk by, and someone drunk with or without dry blood on their face, head or clothes. Without fail there will be lots of people looking absolutely fine, playing on their phones, smoking or chatting outside.

A quick visit to the changing room, followed by a visit to the kitchen to leave our food in the fridge. By the way, the state of the staff kitchen in any hospital is so disgusting that it is easy to understand why we are pretty much immune to every food poisoning bug that there is. Word documents on the walls, with letters in bold and capitalised, reminding us to clean up after ourselves as our mothers don't work here, make you want to make an even bigger mess. The state of the changing room varies from hospital to hospital: from the ones well equipped with at least a shower and a toilet, to those where you freeze in winter and are at risk of having heat stroke in the summer.

Now we enter the department and let whoever is in charge that day know, to make sure all staff that are scheduled for the shift have arrived. Presentism, as the opposite of absenteeism, is common in the NHS. We are told that if we have any symptoms of gastroenteritis or infective illnesses, respiratory or otherwise, we should stay at home. Having said that, being short of only one member of staff really affects waiting times and the workload of the rest. So, I have to say, we do have a dilemma when feeling a bit under the weather.

We look at the list of patients, and then assign ourselves to the next patient waiting to be seen on whichever software system that particular hospital uses. Cubicles are usually occupied by patients that need to receive treatment, be monitored or are not safe to be left elsewhere due to, commonly, dementia. The drunk and intoxicated also do take their share of trolleys. So before calling our first patient in, we have to ask the Nurse in Charge (**NIC**) for a cubicle, a chair or somewhere ranging from the corridor to the cleaner's utility room in order to have a place to see them. Whatever precious space is available is usually reserved for those patients that are being offloaded from ambulances and require a cubicle. Coming to hospital by ambulance, against common belief, does not automatically qualify you to be assigned a cubicle and does not mean that you'll be seen immediately. Most ambulance attendances are redirected to the waiting room, which makes you question whether the use of that mode of transportation was appropriate. See my previous book for further details.

So there we are, with a patient's notes in our hands and no space to see them. In the meantime, we are expected to be moving patients, whether we have a space to examine them or not. Quantity, as it seems, takes priority over quality. If the NIC is competent, they will shuffle patients around to create space. If the NIC, however, is someone who can't be bothered, that was promoted to their senior position, one step at a time, due to the lack of competition and the number of years served rather than because of personal merit, then there is not much help to be expected from them. Even shit floats to the top, as they say.

So we start looking for a suitable place, which can be more or less difficult depending on what we know about our patient from reading the triage notes. If it is something like abdominal or chest pain, then we need a trolley to allow for a proper examination. If it is what sounds like a chest or throat infection, then a chair, or even standing somewhere more or less private to have the chest listened to would be acceptable, although a full examination of the patient, which we are expected to do in pretty much every case that is not a sprain or a fracture, will not be possible, as you cannot examine an abdomen properly with the patient standing or sitting. Keep this in mind for later.

Finally, we find a more or less suitable place, so we go to the waiting room to call our patient. No answer. Lots of enquiring faces, but no answer from the patient in question. A young lady with a canula in her arm stands up from a wheelchair after taking a selfie and walks around the waiting room with her phone raised to the ceiling, searching for signal to upload her photo to her Instagram account. So after a few unanswered calls, we walk outside to see if the patient is there. I mean, where else do you get this service? As far as I know, if I go to a place where I have to wait to be called in, government run or not, I better pay attention. But in the ED, we go the extra mile and look for patients outside. We even look for patients in the toilets, for fuck's sake. But no luck, so we walk back in, leave the notes aside to call them later, and move on, picking up another set of notes and starting all over again. With a bit of luck, the space we have found to see the previous patient in will still be available, but if not, we are back to square one.

After sorting out the next patient, a fortysomething year old male punched in the face several times by a pimp after wanting to have intercourse with a prostitute even though he had only paid for a quick blowjob, at 8 in the morning on his way to work, I go back to call the missing patient again, and do that up to 3 times, despite all the time that is wasted in doing so. And by time wasted, I mean our time. I don't think it is too much to ask that if anyone leaves because they cannot be bothered to wait, or because they are feeling better, they could at least have the decency to let us know instead of taking up our time looking for them. If they don't do it for us, at least they could do it for the others that are waiting to be seen. Like in any other place, we could call patients and if they don't respond, tough luck, but no, this is the NHS, so we have to call people 3 times before taking them off the system and officially discharging them. Because we have to give a fuck even for those that don't give a fuck about us, or others for that matter. Call me a genius if you like, but there is a very easy solution: an LED display like those used in GP Surgeries. Then we can call patients that way and remove them from the system if they have not answered in a predetermined time. It will make the process quicker and more effective, plus they are not expensive: I have done a quick search and they can be found for less than a grand, which is nothing to a Trust which counts its budget in the tens of millions. Another great addition would be to request, like when checking in to a hotel, a credit card deposit. No money taken, but a fine if anyone leaves the department without checking themselves out. Full payment for the ambulance trip, if that was the way they arrived at the ED and left before being seen.

The boy who cried wolf (reloaded)

As you may know from reading my previous book, I am a great believer of involving patients in their treatment and together deciding on the best course of action. I completely respect a patient's informed decisions, whether that means agreeing to a treatment that may have little effect or refusing a lifesaving one. However, I am not here so people can get an x-ray, or antibiotics, or a jab because they think they know best while the responsibility for requesting or prescribing such investigations or treatments lays not on them but on myself. Medical degrees do not grow on trees, and it takes a great deal of knowledge, experience and responsibility to be able to prescribe treatments and request investigations that involve, for example, ionising radiation. If it was as easy as wanting something and ordering it, hospitals would have self-service machines like in McDonalds. When I see a solicitor, it is to ask for legal advice, and not to tell them how they should apply the law. When it comes to the NHS, there are those who seem to believe that they know better than a qualified doctor or practitioner.

Recently, I saw a patient that made me muse on how to accurately convey the complexities we face when dealing with complex patients, when these complexities are not clinical. I have already discussed the topic of crying wolf in my previous book, but this case is an excellent example of everything that is wrong with the way patients have been allowed to take control of what needs to happen.

Female, 32, had a knee injury 3 years ago at work and has been off-sick ever since. Attends because she is still in pain, according to the triage notes. On taking a history from her, before even saying why she sought medical attention today, she relates how initially her injury was missed and she kept coming back in pain to be sent back home, and nobody took her seriously and put her pain down to anxiety, which she had been diagnosed with and was on treatment for. Her companion's attitude, the way he repeats back everything that is said, is that of *you are all shit*. Eventually her GP referred her to orthopaedics outpatients, I suspect more to get rid of her rather than because of clinical need. An MRI showed absolutely nothing, but she kept complaining of pain. Pain is one thing we have no detectors for. If someone says they are in pain, we can think that there is no explanation for or no reason why, but we cannot absolutely rule it out in the same way that we cannot prove wrong a person that claims they have suddenly lost their vision in both eyes. Not in the way that we can prove that someone is not anaemic, hasn't got a fever, or has not broken a bone, anyway. In the case of the vision loss, every test relies on the person reading letters or identifying shapes, so if a malingerer says they cannot see, there is no simple way of scientifically proving they are bullshitting us.

Back to the lady with the normal MRI. You would think that if a pain, or a symptom for that matter, is thoroughly investigated and no reason is found to explain said symptom or pain, you would stop there and then. But not in the NHS. In the NHS the patient says she is in pain, and we all have to believe her. Because she kept complaining of pain she was referred to a knee specialist, and an ultrasound showed, again, nothing. So, even though she is convinced that:

a. there is something seriously wrong with her knee, and
b. there is an ongoing global conspiracy to deny her the right diagnosis and treatment,

she keeps attending the ED to give anyone that sees her the *you-are-all-shit* attitude based on her above beliefs. Why she keeps attending escapes me. That is like going back to a restaurant that gave you a shit meal and service. If I was her and I was convinced of points a and b above, I would go private, get the right diagnosis and treatment, and then sue the NHS motherfuckers that kept me in pain for so long, demanding a huge compensation for my troubles. Returning to the ED, giving abuse, expecting that this time something will be found when all the tests have been negative is plain stupid. But she knows the tests are right, that's why she does not seek help elsewhere.

This time, after my assessment, I discharged her again as I found no cause for her pain. So, considering that she is not epileptic nor has a history of seizures, she decides to have a fit so she is rushed again into the ED, put on a Resus trolley and a myriad of tests are organised. In terms of resources this includes blood tests, a CT scan of her head, urine and pregnancy tests, cardiac monitoring and occupying a cubicle for several hours. A cubicle that could've been used for an ill patient. And, back to the complexities I mentioned earlier, this is what I really want you to understand: if a 32-year-old patient not known to be epileptic has a seizure, it needs to be taken seriously, as nasty things like strokes, brain infections and brain tumours are the usual culprits. Having said that, the probability of an unhappy customer having any of these illnesses resulting in a seizure coinciding with having just been discharged, are probably in the region of a few billions to 1. The likely diagnosis is a functional seizure, also called pseudo seizures which have nothing to do with epilepsy and a lot to do with mental health. Spoiler alert, all the tests for seizures came back negative, which proves the point I am trying to make. This patient's pain is, as diagnosed from the beginning, related to her mental health issues, regardless of what she thinks is causing it.

If the system was designed to minimise unnecessary interventions incurring unnecessary costs, based on probabilities, this patient would be told to either accept that her knee problems are related to her mental health and seek help accordingly, or to fuck off and go waste somebody else's time. This patient would also be denied any further assistance for her knee pain and even be given warnings about the abuse she and her relatives give for free to everyone on every occasion. She has been thoroughly investigated, referred to specialists and reviewed and nothing organic has been found. But because the system does not apply the wisdom of Aesop's fable, she keeps coming back.

I want my taxes, as I'm sure you do too, to be spent fairly, on people that need treatment, or investigations, or whatever the NHS can provide to make them better. Patients like these are a clear waste of time, money and resources for everyone, and believe me when I say that they make us grow a shield around us that ultimately ends up affecting you, the responsible and sensible NHS user.

To err is human

To Err Is Human, wrote the English poet Alexander Pope in his 1711 poem *An Essay on Criticism, Part II*. To err is, in fact, just a matter of sheer numbers. The more patients a doctor sees, or a nurse treats, the greater the chances of erring. I am confident enough to say that there is not a single person that has ever been alive that has never made a mistake in whatever profession they practiced, or in their personal lives, for that matter. It is just that the repercussions of the errors are of differing magnitude according to who makes them. The iconic French Chef Paul Bocuse explained it perfectly when he said "If an architect makes a mistake, he grows ivy to cover it; if a cook makes a mistake, he covers it with some sauce and says it is a new recipe; if a doctor makes a mistake, he covers it with soil." After covering their mistakes with sauces or growing ivy, architects and chefs can continue making plans for new builds or new recipes, and their sleep is not disturbed at night. The price of the soil we have to use to cover our errors, the consequences of making a mistake for a doctor are having to face not only what it means for someone devoted to saving lives to have lost one and the grief caused to the deceased person's relatives, a doctor also has to face the General Medical Council and may lose their license to practice. Although to err is human, a doctor is not allowed to err even once.

"I am only human" was what the disgraced and celebrity wanna-be Matt Hancock said to justify the failures in his management of the Sars-Cov-2 pandemic. Thousands died or suffered, and will continue to die and suffer, as a result of his failures. And as far as I know, he has not been held accountable and nothing financially or professionally has changed for him. Had he been a doctor whose actions led to the death or suffering of even only a few, he would not be allowed to practice ever again and perhaps would even end up in prison.

Remember when I mentioned the inability to perform a proper examination when there were no trolleys available? Very rarely a medical error is due to a single person's incompetence. Many professionals are involved in a patient's care, working together as a safety net. As an example, if a person is to have emergency surgery for a broken limb, a consent form must be signed, which will specify the procedure, the limb to be operated on, and the potential complications. The skin on that limb will then be marked, literally, with a permanent marker, an arrow in black ink pointing to the operation site. On arrival to theatre, the staff will carry out further checks to ensure that the consent form is for the right patient, the correct limb and the correct procedure. The surgeon will also check that he is operating on the correct patient and limb before proceeding. I know that we have all heard the case of someone that got the wrong kidney removed and I can only think of tribalism and diva surgeons, toxic teams and working environments with lack of communication, like those mentioned in my previous book, as the causes for these colossal errors to be allowed to happen.

To Err Is Human asserts that the problem is not bad people in health care, but rather that good people are working in bad systems that need to be made safer. If we miss something for not performing a full examination, it will be completely our fault. Management, the GMC, or the Coroner, will not give a shit about the conditions in which we had to see our patient. It will be deemed a doctor's error, rather than considering all the steps that led to that particular patient not being examined properly or whatever circumstances aligned to achieve such an unfortunate end. That doctor, or that nurse for that matter, depending on the severity of the error and its consequences, will be investigated and even suspended. The system that allowed that error to happen is rarely questioned, therefore preventing any improvements of any kind from being made. Killing the messenger does not solve the problem, it just kills another messenger in a system that cannot really afford to kill any more messengers. The blaming culture prevails over the learning-from-mistakes culture, and as a result, nothing really changes for the better (more on this in the next chapter).

We also have to take into account the fact that, as already mentioned, medicine is not mathematics. That's why we occasionally get it wrong. What you read in the papers is *Man dies after being sent home from hospital* but what they don't tell you is that the man in question presented with dental pain for 2 days which turned out to be caused by a heart attack. If you search for the symptoms of a heart attack, if you are lucky, you might find dental pain mentioned and people don't go to the dentist with tooth pain and get immediately sent to hospital with a suspected heart attack. Equally, I've seen one person presenting with pain in one wrist, nothing else, also having a heart attack. A heart attack in someone presenting with dental or wrist pain does not rank high on the list of possible diagnoses, so anyone unlucky enough to suffer from anything that gives them weird or very unusual symptoms may be unlucky enough not to have a correct diagnosis. This is not the clinician's fault: it is a challenging presentation disguised as a nothing to worry about problem. One hundred percent of doctors will get presentations like these wrong, at least initially. This is what is meant by the expression *shit happens*.

You may also see in the papers, *Teenager died of sepsis after not being given antibiotics in hospital*. What you are not told is that said teenager had haemolytic uraemic syndrome (HUS), a deadly bacterial infection that is made even more lethal by giving antibiotics. It can take between 18 hours and 7 days for the results of bacterial cultures to rule out HUS to be available, depending on the bacteria involved in the infection. So if HUS is suspected, antibiotics must be withheld until ruled out by the culture results, but if the patient dies while waiting for those results, it is not the doctor's or anyone's fault. Again, shit happens. Like dying by being hit by a falling tree or lightning. Although in retrospect, as a way of blaming someone, all fingers will point to the clinician involved in the care of the dead patient.

So what about that for another proposed treatment? How about looking in depth at every mistake or near miss, taking into consideration every aspect of what lead to an error? The Swiss Cheese Model of Accident Causation is a model used in risk analysis and risk management. It illustrates that no accident or error is due to a single cause. It likens systems to multiple slices of Swiss Cheese, you know, the one with holes in it, in which serious adverse consequences take place if all the holes in the slices align, allowing the harm, portrayed in the model as an arrow, to happen. Any intervention with just one of the slices that takes a single hole out of the alignment needed for the arrow to pass through will result in the harm not being done, the error not being committed, the accident never happening. Focusing on only one of the slices, namely the doctor or the nurse, will not stop the same harm, accident or error from ever reoccurring again. But that is usually what happens as you might've already deduced from reading my previous book.

So back to quoting Alexander Pope, *To Err Is Human; to Forgive, Divine.*

The fucking GMC

There is a consensus amongst doctors that the GMC, the regulatory body that we all have to be registered with if we want to practice in the UK, is there to fuck us. Hence the title of this chapter. And all for the affordable price of £420 per year.

The General Medical Council, more commonly known as the GMC, was established in the 1850s as the General Council of Medical Education and Registration of the United Kingdom. Prior to its birth under the Medical Act, there were 19 bodies regulating the medical profession at a local level and with different tests for competence. Its original roles included taking charge of registration, medical education across the UK, publication of a list of available drugs and the directions for their use. The first national medical register was published in 1859.

According to www.legislation.gov.uk, the over-arching objective of the General Medical Council in exercising their functions is the protection of the public. The quest by the GMC to achieve their over-arching objective involves the pursuit of the following goals: a) to protect, promote and maintain the health, safety and well-being of the public; b) to promote and maintain public confidence in the medical profession; and c) to promote and maintain proper professional standards and conduct for members of that profession.

Nothing wrong with these objectives, apart from the fact that they do fuck all about the first and the second. It is comforting for the general public, even for physicians, to know that there is a body overlooking the whole medical profession to avoid people coming to harm due to malpractice or lack of care, in a similar way that it is nice to know that there are food kitchens feeding those in need, or Health & Safety regulations to protect workers from occupational harm.

It was not until fairly recently, in 1995, that the GMC published the first edition of Good Medical Practice, a statement about the standards of patient care that doctors must follow. In the early 21st century, scandals such as the failings at Bristol Royal Infirmary and the Harold Shipman case, brought the GMC under the spotlight with criticism for not striking off more doctors. This is like the police being criticised for not arresting more people, or judges being criticised for not sending more people to jail. Judges should send to jail whoever fucking deserves to go to jail, not lots of people just to make the numbers make sense. It was then that the witch hunt began. Hear me out.

To start with, the presumption of innocence when it comes to a GMC investigation is non-existent: once a doctor is reported to the GMC, that doctor is guilty. Its own recommendations state that doctors should be made to feel innocent until proven otherwise, and that they should use neutral, as opposed to accusatory, language, but you can ask anyone that has ever been referred to the GMC how intimidating and accusatory their supposedly neutral language is. Now, this presumption of culpability comes in several forms, from an immediate ban from practice to an accusation that now the doctor has to dispute to prove their innocence. Don't get me wrong: I am all for coming down hard on a doctor that has used their position for any sort of advantage whether financial, personal or sexual; whose practice falls consistently below standards; that has maliciously removed the wrong kidney or prescribed a treatment that is harmful to their patient; that has unnecessarily chopped off a limb as a result of poor care or improper planning. I am not in favour, however, of treating anyone like a criminal just because someone has accused them of being one.

You might think I am a moron, but I do actually believe in this thing called justice.

To make things worse, a doctor that has been referred to the GMC must now let their employers know, regardless of whether the doctor has done anything wrong or not, and if looking for a new job, the doctor must also disclose this in the application, before any conclusions or verdicts have even been reached. As if being investigated by the GMC does not sound serious or dodgy or anything. Like any member of the public being falsely accused and having to explain to their potential employer that they are not guilty, but nonetheless they are under investigation because someone has accused them of stealing from their previous employer. That will definitely win them some brownie points at the interview.

An article published in the International Business Times in December 2015 discusses how the way the GMC deals with doctors is like "hard-wiring cruelty into the NHS", especially for vulnerable professionals, those suffering from mental health or addiction problems; how doctors can become marginalised with little support, and how they invariably felt, surprise surprise, guilty until proven otherwise. The article mentions cases where the investigation dragged on for as long as 5 years, with the consequent loss of families, homes, livelihoods, and even lives, with 28 doctors committing suicide while under investigation for malpractice between 2005 and 2013, one doctor leaving a suicide note reading "I am extremely stressed and cannot carry on like this. I hold the GMC responsible for making my condition worse with no offer of help." Was anyone in the GMC arrested for this death? My arse they were. Did anything change in the way the GMC operates? My arse, again.

In the GMC's quest to strike off more professionals, the number of doctors undergoing fitness to practice investigations has risen drastically by 54% since 2010. But despite the rise, more than 80% of cases result in no action being taken against the doctor, leading to calls for the system to be reformed, while fuck all is done about it, as usual. Professor Louise Appleby, an independent expert from the University of Manchester who in 2015 lead the GMC's review of its own fitness to practice procedures, has questioned the number of investigations conducted each year, saying there are too many for the number of doctors registered in the UK. The review concluded that complaints against doctors "may do more overall harm than good in terms of patient care", as the majority of doctors who are reported to the GMC are found to have no significant case to answer. But the GMC, anally, insists that it is required by law to investigate.

    Often I hear at work let's do this or that other test "just to cover our backs." That is an expression I detest. I always tell junior doctors and nurses that as long as we do what is best for the patient under the circumstances, and follow the advice set out in protocols and guidelines, we do not need *to cover our backs*. When doing my research to write this chapter I realised how wrong I have been. When a doctor is referred to the GMC, especially in high profile cases like that of Dr Hadiza Bawa-Garba (which I will discuss further later on), and the case is covered by the media and/or when a child dies, the GMC will try to cover its own back and not be criticised, as admitted by them on their web page, for not striking off more doctors. Suddenly, medicolegal documents and fair trials are no longer important, only the reputation of the GMC. A parallel case with parallel events, as opposed to what is documented and actually happened, is considered, and doctors are investigated based on those alternative versions of events. In retrospect, it is easy to criticise, and impartiality is lost. Let me give you an example: a child attends the ED with a head injury. The child is seen by a doctor and on examination, nothing is found that causes concern. There is no indication to proceed with CT scanning of the head, which by the way, is a huge amount of radiation for a child's brain and must not be considered lightly. Remember that the easy option for a doctor is to scan every head, but by doing so, the doctor is also increasing the chances of that child developing a brain tumour in the future as a consequence of the radiation received. Remember also that under the *Ionising Radiation (Medical Exposure) Regulations 2017*, we are responsible and accountable for any radiation we expose our patients to, which must be clearly justified. Benefits must always justify risks. So without any indications to proceed with any scanning, the child is observed for a few hours, continues to show no worrying signs and is discharged with head injury advice, usually a leaflet, for parents to bring the child back to the ED if anything changes. The child goes home, starts vomiting or goes drowsy. The child is brough back to the ED, is seen by a doctor, worrying signs are now present and consequently the child is sent for a CT head, as the suspicion of a bleed is now high. The child is diagnosed with a bleed, goes into a coma and dies a week or 2 later. There is absolutely nothing wrong with what doctors have done for this child. But the parents now say their child was not carefully reviewed before discharge and they were not given an advice leaflet, even though these details are clearly documented in the notes. At the Coroner's inquest, it will be decided that the doctor failed to appreciate the seriousness of the injury and should not have discharged the patient. We all know that illuminating expertise and wisdom that hindsight provides. At the GMC investigation it will be decided that documenting that the child was fit to be discharged was not appropriate because, duh, the child had a bleed and died. The doctor, who has followed the best practice guidelines to the letter, might be banned from practicing again, or given a warning, not to mention the stress, the financial burden and the damage to that doctor's reputation. Any doctor would have proceeded in the same way, but this time, as the saying goes, shit did happen. People die while in surgery, or during a hospital admission, but that does not mean that it is anybody's fault. The hospital, however, and specially the GMC will always prefer a scapegoat to *an act of god*, as insurance companies call it when they refuse to pay for damages. A perfectly capable doctor, if still allowed to practice, will start from now on practicing defensive medicine, which means lowering the bar to scan children's heads and referring for admission, effectively passing on the responsibility to someone else. Are those children given a higher risk of cancer? Yes. Are these patients going to take a bed unnecessarily? Of course. But is the doctor going to get in trouble with the GMC again for not doing what was not indicated in the first place? Nopedy nope. And this is how putting patients first turns into saving my arse first. That's how caring about all aspects of patient's health becomes not giving a shit. That's how the doctor-patient relationship becomes a doctor-potentialtroublewiththeGMC relationship. And as you can imagine, the situation does not benefit anyone, not the resources available, nor the doctor, nor the patient. I am sure this is what Professor Appleby means by "may do more overall harm than good in terms of patient care". Just look at the amount of negative tests patients have these days, the number of unnecessary admissions, and the state of the NHS.

You may think that doctors have patient's lives on their hands, and therefore, extraordinary measures and procedures must be followed to not allow any harm. And I would agree with you, but other factors must be taken into account and considered when potentially ruining the lives and livelihoods of innocent and perfectly capable practitioners. Anyone can literally see a doctor with a complaint that requires an intimate examination, be seen with a chaperone and then accuse the doctor of touching inappropriately denying that a chaperone was present. Even if this is all documented and the chaperone testifies that they were present and nothing unprofessional happened, the doctor will be referred to the GMC, and it will take months to investigate the case while the doctor is, in all likelihood, suspended from work. It may well be concluded at the end that there was no wrongdoing but think of that doctor's reputation and even family: "Honey, I have been accused of touching a female patient inappropriately, but it is not true. However, I am not allowed to work from now on and I am going to be investigated for it." Which partner, girlfriend, boyfriend or spouse would not be affected by such an accusation? And if that wasn't enough, being investigated by the GMC, even if nothing was found, has to now be declared in every job application. Again, brownie points galore. Put yourself in that situation and imagine what your life would be like if you had been falsely accused of any crime, found innocent, but then had to carry that label, disclosing it to your employer and any potential future employers, for the foreseeable future.

In the same way, a doctor's responsibility is so huge that I find it hard to think of any other profession that can be compared. We are respectable and responsible members of society, although that is only when it comes to responsibilities, not when it comes to perks. If a judge mistakenly sentences an innocent person to jail, little trouble comes the judge's way. If you ask me, I'd much rather have a kidney removed unnecessarily than spend 10 years of my life in jail. Yet, the treatment that the professionals responsible for those 2 errors receive is not even close to comparable. I hope you get the point that I am trying to make.

But then, as respectable and responsible members of society, as I said, we get no perks, no advantages whatsoever. As a doctor, you don't get a loan or a mortgage easier than anyone else; you are not treated better or given any complimentary drinks on a plane for being there in case anything happens, even if you have attended to someone that felt ill during the flight (and I know this from personal experience); your word is not more valid than your accuser's, even if you have documented in that patient's notes, which is effectively a medico-legal document, what you are defending. If a doctor gets involved in a fight, even if it is in self-defence, the GMC will be on the doctor's back like lightning. If a doctor is caught drink driving, even on their days off, mama GMC will get the doctor by the balls. There are doctors that have got into trouble with the GMC for being involved with prostitutes while on holiday abroad, for fuck's sake. And no, I do not know any of these latter examples from personal experience. So, as you can see, a doctor is treated like everybody else but expected to behave better than everybody else, not only at work, but all the fucking time. With zero benefits in return. Nice, innit?

I would love it if it was like that for everybody: that plumber that left a leak when installing my new basin that I cannot get hold of now while the stains keep getting bigger on my ceiling; the company that installed my new windows, some of which do not seal properly, that I have been chasing to come and sort them out for months on end; the mechanic that forgot to tighten a few bolts and as a result someone died in a car crash, all reported to their regulatory bodies and banned from work with immediate effect. Anyone that has suffered due to any trades' cowboys will perfectly understand what I am talking about.

Now, back to my point. I feel, and so do many of the doctors I know, that the GMC is not adapting to the times or the new challenges of the system and demands of the service users, and therefore is no longer fit to regulate today's doctors. Just remember the conditions we have to work in described in previous chapters. The GMC is, I want to believe, well aware of this, but still approaches every referral as if we worked in perfect, flawless, adequate environments where everything runs smoothly like clockwork. The GMC does not understand the pressures, the abuse, both verbal and physical, that staff are subjected to, not only from patients but from managers and even colleagues; the exhaustion, the lack of job satisfaction that, whether we like it or not, influences our relationships with other members of staff and with patients. We are not robots, nor are we tin men: we have feelings and all of the above takes its toll. We cannot just reset how we feel and start from scratch with the next patient. I would love for representatives of the GMC to be present routinely in ED departments around the country to have a feel for what really is happening and to realise how unrealistic their expectations of how a doctor should behave are. They could pay regular visits, unannounced and undercover, of course, not like the visits from the Care Quality Commission (CQC), known well in advance so extra members of staff can be hired for that day, and everything can be staged to please them and pass their inspections. Only to go back to the same shit that it was as soon as they are gone. Funny thing is that departments and Trusts know what their flaws are, because they effectively correct them for the CQC visits. It begs the question why are these flaws allowed to perpetuate themselves?

Jack Adcock, a 6-year-old Down's syndrome little boy with a chronic and congenital heart condition died hours after being admitted into Leicester Royal Infirmary in 2011. Dr Hadiza Bawa-Garba, the paediatric Registrar on duty that day, was responsible for the paediatric cover of various wards, including maternity and the ED, as well as taking GP calls referring patients or asking for advice.

On top of that, she was also covering for another paediatric Registrar, who according to different sources, either did not turn up or was on a training course that day, usually booked well in advance, but no cover had been arranged. Dr Bawa-Garba had just returned from a 14-month maternity leave and was working in an unfamiliar hospital having received no induction, which I can safely say is usually the norm. To add to the failures of that tragic day, the IT system was down, which meant she had to telephone the labs for urgent blood results, and due to the amount of extra work she had to do, there were delays in checking both blood results and x-rays. She had also discussed the child at handover with the paediatric Consultant on-call that day who, despite having been made aware of the case, chose not to review the 6-year-old.

Yet, Dr Bawa-Garba was made the scapegoat (see the pattern?) and was given full responsibility for the death of Jack Adcock. She was convicted of manslaughter on the grounds of gross negligence in November 2015 and was suspended from practice for 12 months by an independent tribunal. The GMC, however, appealed that decision, wanting to get her permanently struck off the medical register, arguing that the doctor contributed to the little boy's death. No consideration was given to all the other contributing factors that the hospital had failed to rectify. The ruling and the GMC's position sparked outcry from doctors in Britain who saw reflected the environment that they have to work in and therefore realised that this same thing could, at any time, happen to any of them. Thousands of doctors crowdfunded more than £300,000 to help Dr Bawa-Garba fund an appeal, gaining so much support that even the then Health Secretary, Jeremy Hunt ordered a review of the case and the laws applied. In 2018 Dr Bawa-Garba won the appeal against the GMC's decision to strike her off for good, the fucking regulatory body that should be fit to carry out such proceedings with fairness. The GMC had to give her her registration number back. She completed her specialist training and gained consultant status in April 2022. Had it not been for the support of so many fellow colleagues and the crowdfunding money to fund her appeal, a perfectly good doctor with an unblemished record and committed to good medical practice would have had her life ruined by the very organisation that is supposed to be guiding doctors. The GMC should really concentrate its efforts on dealing with doctors who are dishonest, deliberately and repeatedly, rather than those who are conscientious and are involved in a single error.

Once again, this is how it works: the system is faulty but, like in the case of the whistle-blowers I discussed in my previous book, someone is sacrificed, usually a hardworking and perfectly competent doctor, and nothing changes. The blame is washed off of the faulty system, the GMC avoids criticism for not striking off more doctors, and the family of the unfortunate victim is happy that someone has been made to pay, usually with statements like "we do not want what happened to our son to happen to anybody else" or "justice has been done" when in reality, nothing, absolutely nothing has changed. The death of their relative has changed nothing, other than taking a sacrificial lamb, a perfectly good doctor, out of the profession. When the next tragedy happens, the whole charade is repeated again. I can guarantee that a doctor can show up for a night shift in the ED to find out that no one else has turned up, be expected to still do the job, and if a patient dies that night from an avoidable cause, the doctor will be made the scapegoat. Not the system, but the doctor.

So, to make a final statement, I hope it has become clear that the GMC is no longer fit for purpose. On top of that, High Courts and Employment Tribunals have ruled against the GMC in several cases of racism, and concluded in one of them that the GMC was "looking for material to support allegations against [the doctor], rather than fairly assessing materials presented." It is also being sued, with the support of the British Medical Association (BMA), by the widow of a senior consultant anaesthetist who took his own life after being informed by the GMC that he would be investigated for inappropriately touching a teenage girl to whom he had administered sedatives, known to cause hallucinations, for a dental procedure. And don't get me wrong, I am all for the law to act against those who abuse their position, but I am also a defender of the status of innocence until proven otherwise. To show the extremes the GMC will go to in order to exert its power and elude responsibility, an article published in the Mail Online on the 23rd March 2023 under the headline *EXCLUSIVE: Great Ormond Street children's doctor is suspended from NHS job for six months... for using his wife's free TFL travel pass*, discusses how a consultant paediatric cardiac anaesthetist at Great Ormond Street Hospital (GOSH) was suspended for 6 months from putting to sleep for surgery children that needed heart operations. His heinous crime, using his wife's free travel pass for which after being caught he paid around £800 in fines and compensation costs, lead the GMC to suspend him from his extremely specialised job, with the subsequent disruption to sick children's heart surgery, because his actions "represented a significant breach of GMC's code, which states: 'You must make sure that your conduct justifies your patient's trust in you and the public's trust in the profession.'"

But it seems the GMC does not apply the same standards to itself. On the 15th March 2023 a British Medical Journal (BMJ) investigation under the headline *GMC is criticised for investments in Nestlé and McDonald's* reported that the regulator had direct investments in fast food companies, like McDonald's, or corporations such as Nestlé and Astra Zeneca. The report goes on to say that, I quote, "doctors have criticised the investments because of the link between fast food and soft drink companies' products and rising rates of obesity worldwide and because the investments are not published on the GMC's website." After this report, I quote again, "the GMC is also considering publishing its investments on its website after The BMJ pointed out that they were not displayed transparently." So how is that for fulfilling the over-arching objectives of protecting, promoting and maintaining professional standards, public health, and public confidence in the profession? How is that for lack of transparency and accountability to its members? It would be like the catholic church investing in abortion clinics. Another case of do as I say, not as I do.

And yet there is no hashtag about it on twitter, or any campaigns to seriously demand accountability, or call for action against or to reform the GMC. Such is the level of fear amongst doctors, feeling powerless against such a Goliath. The time has come to stand against the tyranny of the GMC, to strike perhaps by refusing to pay our registration fees, all doctors at once, and create a brand-new regulatory body that is fair, that takes the side of its registered doctors until proven guilty, like in any other country of the world. If you are a doctor and feel identified after reading this chapter, please get in touch. If we get together, in enough numbers, we might be able to change something.

Stepping into my shoes (Part 2)

After all the time wasted looking for a patient that wasn't there, well, that actually was there but left without telling anyone, I have picked up the next patient's notes and while I am looking at the triage notes *31-year-old, female, attends with abdominal pain for several days,* vitals within normal range… the phone rings. Phones in the ED are for us to reach someone or another department. If anyone wants to reach our department, whether internally or externally, they call the NIC station's phone. Our phones are not supposed to ring on their own unless we have paged someone. Accordingly, most members of staff, whose job is not to pick up the phone, are reluctant to do so. However, after much ringing and some hesitation from my part, I pick it up and identify myself to the caller as one of the ED doctors. It is a relative enquiring about her mother, a patient I know nothing about. However, I sympathise with this worried daughter and check on the computer to try to gather more info: a surgical patient, directly referred by her GP to the surgical team. Nothing to do with us, although she's in the department because that is where the surgical team asked the GP to send the patient to be seen by them, rather than directly to the Surgical Assessment Unit. Even so, I want to be helpful, so I go and pick up this patient's notes and have a quick browse through. I ask the relative what it is that she is after, within the confidentiality terms of engagement. She wants to know why her mother is still in the department after

8 hours since arrival. She is demanding to be told why she has not been moved to the ward yet. I politely let her know that all I can see written in the notes is that she is awaiting senior surgical review before a decision is made regarding further management. "You must be fucking kidding me!" is her reply. I, again politely, let her know that I am not kidding her, just reading what someone from the team looking after her mother has written in the notes in the PLAN section. "You are a doctor. Why can you not review her and make a fucking decision?" is the response I get. Now, I understand the frustration for the delays and all that, but I was minding my own business, happened to be sitting by the phone when it rang, and answered it to be helpful. Instead, I get rudeness and abuse. I could've let it ring to boredom. My patient is still waiting to be called in the WR. It's not like I had nothing to do and decided to try my luck as a telephone helpline operator. By this time, I decide to be a little bit firmer and I, again, politely, repeat to this relative that I have already explained that her mother is not an ED patient and therefore has nothing to do with us, and certainly nothing to do with me in particular. We only get involved with patients that are not ED patients if they deteriorate whilst in the department. Otherwise, our nurses do nurse them, but that's about it. The relative tells me that she finds it hard to believe that I know nothing about her mother, that what kind of care is that, and she asks for my name to make a complaint. At this point I cannot give a fuck. I tell her that I was just trying to help, that her mother is already being looked after by the surgical team and that I am not giving her my name. She starts shouting something about going to the newspapers and heads are going to roll and I just put the phone down, take a few breaths, remind myself that this is precisely why hospital phones that ring on their own must be regarded as possessed by one of Satan's minions, and make a mental note-to-self to never answer the phone, ever, again. So if you ever need to phone an ED to enquire about a relative and no one picks up, now you know why. Spare a thought for the ungrateful cunts that have taught us to ignore ringing phones into oblivion.

I stand up and, after going through all of the usual enquiries to find a free cubicle, I am assigned one that has just been vacated. I go to check if it is ready and I find blood-stained sheets, blankets and a gown still on the trolley, a bedside table with a half drunk cup of tea, biscuit crumbs, and the cherry on top of the cake: a urine bottle, full of urine, left in the sink. I put some gloves on, clear the mess, and wipe the trolley clean. I go to get some clean sheets for the trolley and by the time I come back, ignoring the you-have-to-ask-the-NIC-for-a-space rule, one of the surgeons is walking a patient to the cubicle I have just cleaned. "Yo yo yo", I cry. The surgeon tries to persuade me, promising it will only take 5 minutes to examine her patient, but I know their tricks. So after much huffing and puffing by the surgeon, I make my way to the WR to finally call my patient.

While I am negotiating my way through the trolleys, chairs and relatives occupying the corridors, the emergency alarm goes off. The emergency alarm is that alarm that is triggered by pulling the red button, or rather a red triangle thingy, on the wall of the cubicle. It means that a member of staff needs urgent help, and its annoyingly loud sound can be heard all over the ED. A display, usually by the NIC's station, shows which cubicle or area the alarm has been triggered from. By then, anyone witnessing the event would be much amused by seeing members of staff stopping what they are doing and looking around, others coming from behind the curtains of the cubicles and then, once the NIC has shouted out where help is needed for everyone to hear while the alarm is still sounding loud, a horde of people start running towards the area or cubicle in question. It is ridiculous, really. A couple of people attending the alarm would suffice, but somehow everyone is compelled to run to help, only to return about 10 seconds later due to it being a false alarm, the knob having been pulled accidentally, as is the case 9 out of 10 times.

My patient, that one whose notes I picked up before I answered the phone, before I had to stop a surgical invasion of the cubicle I had prepared, and before the emergency alarm went off, is still patiently waiting to be called in from the WR, completely oblivious to the exciting adventures of her notes in my back pocket, and probably wondering why other patients that arrived after her have been called in and she is still waiting. I still manage to get stopped 3 times on my way to the WR: once by one of the nurses asking me whether a patient I know nothing about looks well enough to wait in the WR after having been brought in to have an ECG; a second time by another nurse asking me to prescribe analgesia for her patient; and finally by a HCA waving a print-out of a venous blood gas result fresh from the analyser that he needs me to acknowledge by signing it. I know fuck all about these 3 patients, but still sign their results and prescribe analgesia, as requested. This is normal practice in every ED.

I finally make it to the WR, take the notes out of my back pocket and proceed to finally call my patient. On reading her name, I realise that she has a foreign name that I am not sure how to pronounce, so I shout it out pronouncing it as a best guess. The usual faces turning to hear the name. Someone asks from the back of the WR if I am calling a completely different name but, to their credit, it does kind of sound how I pronounced my patient's name, to whom I shake my head side to side in denial. I shout out the name again, this time with a slightly different pronunciation, and again, no response. I want to shout "the woman with the belly pain!", but that would be a breach of confidentiality, so I am about to try again when I see a woman whose estimated aged would coincide with the patient's I am looking for, collecting her belongings and walking towards me. She does not look like someone who has abdominal pain severe enough to attend the ED, confirmed by the fact that she is carrying a McDonalds bag with her and eating a burger as she walks. You see, those first few moments of seeing the patient are particularly important, since they give us, observing clinicians, a lot of valuable information. Although I am sure that in this case even the most inexperienced monkey would've reached the same conclusion. If the triage notes say *injury to ankle* and upon being called the patient walks without a limp, the diagnosis of a sprain, or nothing, is made instantly (you'd be surprised to know that *No Abnormality Found*, is actually a diagnosis frequently used in the ED);

if the notes read *shortness of breath* and the patient is breathing normally while they walk, we know we are not going to find anything of concern in our examination. As a note, it amazes me beyond comprehension being told by a patient that they are short of breath when they are talking in long sentences without having to stop to breathe after every few words. Have these people never run, or been under water long enough to know what being short of breath really feels like?

Back to my patient, I realise that she is also carrying a small suitcase, the type that Ryanair would allow you to take onto the plane. This has actually become quite a regular custom in EDs, patients walking around with a suitcase as if they were going on a yoga retreat or on holiday. So how is that for valuable information? On top of knowing that there cannot be anything of concern for a young female with abdominal pain who does not seem to be in pain and is eating a McDonalds, I also perceive that she is coming determined to be admitted, and possibly also has a list of investigations in mind which of course she has googled beforehand. This is going to be anything but fun.

Weeping blisters and tears

I get the impression that patients feel they are entitled to insult us, shout and swear at us, and even kick us as part of their ED visit experience. Pain seems to be what justifies all of the above. You see, when we examine a painful belly, or a broken limb, some degree of pain is inevitable. Pain also gives us clues as to what the underlying problem might be, so as part of the examination, we do have to explore pain to guide us on how to proceed next. Complaining of abdominal pain tells us, in most cases, only the area we have to focus on, but unless we obtain more information from a detailed history and a thorough examination, we cannot be sure whether it is severe constipation requiring laxatives or a perforated bowel requiring emergency surgery.

Recently I was dealing with a young patient with a catheter that was not draining properly. One of the first things we do is fiddle with it lest the tip is displaced and sitting outside the bladder, namely in the urethra. When I pushed this patient's catheter in, they complained of a lot of pain before letting me know that if I moved the catheter again, they would kick me, and they did not want to do that. What a fucking cunt. I just smiled to myself. According to that logic, if the patient kicks me, it will cause me pain that then will justify me kicking the patient back. As long as I use reasonable force, it will also justify me doing the kicking alleging self-defence.

I think that it all started with mentally disturbed patients being kind of allowed to hit doctors and nurses, but somehow it has extended to every patient that feels a little upset about anything. This is no surprise, as it seems to be the pattern followed by everything else in the NHS, from food and drinks for patients, to transportation from and to the patient's residence, to the way staff are spoken to by patients.

The case I want to discuss in this chapter is that of a teenage female that attended the ED with sore genitals. A junior doctor was dealing with her and came to ask me whether it would be appropriate to do an internal examination. He explained that the patient had developed painful blisters, that were now weeping, in her down below. This is very suggestive of genital herpes, and an internal examination using a vaginal speculum, that piece of equipment shaped like an albatross' beak that is introduced into the vagina, is neither needed nor indicated because, well, it's bloody painful. The junior doctor had never seen genital herpes before, so I asked him to let me have a look first.

He leads me to the room where the patient was, accompanied by her mother and grandmother. After introducing myself and explaining why I was getting involved, I ask for permission to have a look at the affected area and with a simple glance, my suspicion is confirmed. I look at the junior doctor and ask him to refer the patient to gynaecology, for them to review, confirm the diagnosis and treat. Grandmother then asks me what the problem is, to which I respond that they need to wait for the gynaecologist to assess but she ain't having it. She asks me again, and I give her the same response. While the mother is not saying anything, simply looking at me, the grandmother, for the third time, is insisting on being told what the problem is, even if it is just my opinion. I tell her that since she insists to know what I am thinking of, my working diagnosis is genital herpes. The teenager starts crying, her mother starts hugging her and crying with her. The grandmother starts shouting at me that her granddaughter has only had 1, current, boyfriend and that I should not have said it was genital herpes unless I was absolutely sure. I am shocked. What do you respond to that? She is telling me I should've done what I was doing in the first place. I take a few deep breaths and when she stops shouting, I remind her that I did not volunteer any information, and only gave her my opinion, on the understanding that it was just my opinion, after she repeatedly insisted. She still insists in the not-saying-anything-unless-absolutely-sure. I ask her if she will apologise to me if the diagnosis is correct. She shouts she won't. So there you go. I turn around and get the fuck out of the room. I chased the swab results a few days later and it was confirmed: genital herpes. I probably would've got a complaint if it wasn't, blaming me for psychological stress and the anxiety caused. No apology received. Fuck you, grandmother. I hope you get herpes too.

The wrong queue

"I have been waiting for 4 hours and now you tell me you cannot help me." This is a statement that we hear quite frequently, usually with the waiting time exaggerated by an hour or 2. On the case notes we can see exactly the time a patient registered, the time they first saw a nurse in triage and so on, so please stop the bullshit. We know how long someone has been waiting.

Increasingly people attend the ED as a means to bypass the normal way of operating. For example, a woman finds a lump in her breast. The worry, of course, is breast cancer. The normal procedure would be to see her GP for her GP to examine her as soon as possible and if needed, make a referral through the Cancer Pathway in which a specialist review must take place within 2 weeks. What people do instead is attend the ED demanding to have all the necessary tests and consultations to be given a diagnosis on the same day. I can totally understand why that woman would be worried to death, and in a perfect world, that is how things would be, but we live in a far from perfect world, and if we don't understand that, we chisel away whatever hope is left of making it work for all of us. Remember that we go into this profession because we genuinely want to help people, not because we are sadist motherfuckers who enjoy denying patients access to investigations and treatment. Remember also that we are just as neglected as patients are. Recently I had to aspirate a fluid collection in a patient's chest and had to improvise with makeshift tools because the equipment I needed was not in stock. The equivalent of immobilising a fracture with a broom stick and some bandage instead of a Plaster of Paris, if you get my drift. Attending the ED only puts more pressure on the system and makes it worse for those who really need to be seen and investigated as an Emergency. Blaming us for the shortcomings and failures of the system only makes us reconsider why the fuck we do this at all and why on Earth we care about whether patients receive quality care or are seen by a witch doctor.

  On a similar note, a case comes to mind of a child attending the Paediatric ED with his father, who was complaining to us that his child had had nothing to eat for a few hours and was hungry, making it sound as if his son was about to die of starvation. When the nurses told him that food was not provided for children and pointed him out in the direction of the vending machine, suddenly the father was happy for his child to remain hungry. And that was just a few quid for a sandwich, a packet of crisps, a drink and a chocolate bar. This is a recurrent pattern in which it is ok to complain and make demands when it is believed to be the hospital's responsibility, but those demands are suddenly of no importance when the responsibility is transferred back to the complainant. There were, a year or so ago, a few articles in mainstream newspapers discussing new guidance from the National Institute for Health and Care Excellence (**NICE**) which advised against offering strong painkillers to people with arthritis, and instead suggested encouraging patients to take responsibility for their own health by losing weight and doing exercise, both measures proven to improve symptoms of osteoarthritis, as well as helping to regulate blood pressure and blood sugar levels in type 2 diabetics, but good luck with that. In my experience, people much prefer the quick fix, especially when it is provided for them and it does not cost them any extra money.

  People's perception of how serious an injury is, is totally exaggerated. I have seen patients coming with a bandage on their arm, turning their gaze away as I unwrapped it, telling me that it was quite a nasty injury that would require stitches, for me to see a small cut a little deeper than a scratch that I sorted out with a little bit of glue. They wait in ED to be seen for hours because they think their injury is serious. It makes me think that people have lost their common sense. Their knowledge of what a test is for, is pretty much non-existent, and that is precisely why they need a doctor to tell them what they need, to reach a diagnosis. Some patients have a little bump to the head, with no worrying symptoms and come demanding a CT scan of their brains. To order a CT scan, which involves a huge amount of radiation and a significant increase in the risk of developing something nasty in the years to come, we must have at least a good and clear indication that something might be going on inside that person's skull, namely a tumour, a bleed or a fracture. Otherwise, we would be exposing people to unnecessary harmful radiation. Besides, a CT scan costs hundreds of pounds, but that is secondary, and as mentioned before, there are Ionising Radiation Regulations that make the requesting practitioner responsible for the radiation administered to a patient. The NHS will cover the cost of any investigation, procedure or treatment, as long as it is the right thing to do for a suspected condition or presentation. Not because a patient, who thinks that the cause of their headache can be diagnosed with an x-ray, requests it. The NHS will cover everything, and I mean everything, needed to diagnose and treat as long as it is done through the appropriate channels and only if it is indicated. So let me propose another treatment for these cases: when a test, a treatment or a hospital admission is not indicated but the patient still insists on having it, the NHS will offer the option to have it, but it will have to be paid for by the patient, in advance. And in the case of the tests, not only will the patient have to pay for the test, but also for the report of the test, after signing a disclaimer exempting us from any responsibility for the potential harm they may suffer by having that test or investigation done. If we were wrong, the NHS will refund them the money. I think that would be fair. If you have read my previous book, you know how much a hospital admission costs. An extremely popular test, a CT scan, typically costs between £430 and

£907; a Chest X-Ray, between £79 and £140; and a routine blood test around £150 at private hospitals and clinics in the UK. I am sure that by offering this option, the problem will be sorted once and for all. Simple as that.

Now, let me tell you what that overused statement with which I started this chapter means with an example. There are several stages after someone says that, and invariably those stages happen one after the other. Remember that it is not used by people who attend with a heart attack, a stroke or a fractured bone, because we can and actually do help those that attend the ED legitimately with an emergency condition. The example involves a very obese, unemployed man with lower abdominal pain. He is happily texting on his phone when I call him from the WR, but as soon as he realises it's his turn, he starts doing a display of grunts and faces to show how much pain he is in. Too late, mate, I have already seen you.

I take him to the cubicle that I have already reserved for him, which is still free when I wheel him in, because of course, he is in a wheelchair and refuses to walk, and taking his time, grunting and puffing, he transfers to the trolley. After taking a history and examining him, I let him know my opinion, which is that there does not seem to be anything seriously wrong with him (note the *seriously* on that statement), certainly nothing that requires any emergency intervention, and that, however, he should make an appointment to see his own GP to have them look into his pain, perhaps arrange non-urgent investigations to get to the root of it. I offer to prescribe good painkillers until he manages to see his doctor. He is not happy with this. I get the impression he thought I would get him seen by the surgeons as a matter of urgency. He then reminds me that I have a duty of care (DoC) and that if I miss whatever is causing his pain, he will sue me hard. I tell him that I am happy taking that responsibility, as that is part of the contract, but I also let him know that it is not nice to be asked for a professional opinion and then be spoken to like that when the opinion is given. He also tells me, his voice now raised, that he is not happy to have waited 3 hours for me to just send him to his

GP with no further tests, and then the funny story: he tells me that he pays my salary. I was having a very shitty shift, as is becoming the norm, and I allowed myself a bit of time to think twice about whether to go ahead and say what I wanted to say. I finally thought fuck it and went for it. I asked this patient what his job was, to which he responded that he was on benefits. Then, with a huge smile on my face, I told him that not only he did not pay my salary, but it was I who paid his benefits. He did not utter a word after that. He did not expect such a response. These patients are not used to anyone confronting them about their bullshit. I did not say anything that was not true.

I had a mother once telling me that what was wrong with her perfectly healthy child was that little insects had gotten into his blood stream and were biting him from the inside. People that have never had a heart attack telling me that the pain in their chest is like heart attack pain. People walking around in no pain wanting to be scanned for internal bleeding and shit like that. I mentioned in my previous book the case of the young man jerking his legs after having a minor electric shock. Perhaps that is the problem, that we don't challenge enough. That would explain why people attend demanding an x-ray for a headache, or for pains and aches in which doing an x-ray would result in unnecessary radiation with no actual diagnostic benefit whatsoever. It would be like requesting an x-ray to diagnose anaemia. Perhaps it is about time that we do that more often, tell people off for coming at 3am with a pain they have had for months, or for coming to the ED with a non-emergency problem at all. Although that is putting oneself in the line of fire, as telling people things like that inevitably ends in vicious complaints that, somehow, makes us the bad guys. It is weird how law enforcement does not give a shit that you didn't know that what you have done is illegal; how your mortgage provider does not care whether you understand interest rates or not; or even how the tax man has no mercy when claiming money from you when you weren't aware there was a tax you had to pay. When it comes to healthcare, people are not only allowed, but also expected, to be completely ignorant about their own health and their own diseases, so everything they do is justified. They don't even need to know what medication they are on, or even what they take medication for. "It is all in my records" they say. Sometimes patients tell us they have no significant medical history, and it turns out they had chemotherapy for cancer 3 months ago. It is always the doctor's fault, the doctor's responsibility to know about everybody's conditions. "The doctor gave me medication without checking if I was pregnant" said the woman who was late on her period and had not done herself a pregnancy test.

Now, regarding the issue of that DoC that these time wasters mention so often. The DoC refers to practitioners taking reasonable steps to obtain a proper history, to investigate appropriately, to make differential diagnoses, referrals to specialists if indicated and, in a nutshell, take action, provide a course of treatment and arrange follow up if necessary. This basically defines what the duties of a doctor are. We are doctors because we care and because we want to help our patients. We didn't choose this profession because we want to play Russian roulette, harming people and our own careers on the way. This DoC, of course, has to be taken in context: a patient might need a hip replacement due to osteoarthritis, but I am under no obligation to refer him urgently to the orthopaedic team at any time of the day or night to have surgery immediately. The DoC lays with that patient's GP through a referral to the orthopaedic outpatients department. Unless, of course, that hip replacement is needed as an emergency due to a fractured hip. That is different, and I want to believe that anyone can understand that.

I genuinely believe that people think that our DoC involves being their mothers and feeding them when they are hungry, tucking them into bed, and even wiping their arses when they open their bowels. "Sorry doctor, I am hungry, you have a DoC to feed me" or "I need a taxi home, but after a night out I have no money, so you have a DoC to pay for one for me." Some people's concept of what our DoC is seems to extend further than their own DoC for their own health and well-being. I have seen intravenous drug users that have developed endocarditis, an infection of the heart from injecting in unhygienic conditions, have had heart valves replaced to save their lives, and have continued injecting and effectively fucking up the healthy valves they still had. I have seen emphysema patients that rely on supplementary oxygen 24 hours a day smoking happily. But the moment we refuse to treat them any longer unless they take responsibility for their own well-being, we are violating their human rights and neglecting them by breaching our DoC. And that is how the taxes that you pay towards the NHS are utterly wasted on people that don't give a shit about themselves but expect us to.

So back to the title of this chapter, it is not my fault, or anybody's fault for that matter, that a patient has chosen to wait in the wrong queue. Waiting to be seen in ED does not work like a loyalty card that gives people access to more investigations the longer they spend in the WR. If you are flying with EasyJet, no amount of complaining is going to get you checked in at the British Airways desk just because you joined the wrong queue. So please, everybody needs to stop the crap, and play their part if the NHS is to stay afloat. They need to stop blaming us for their own short comings. We can only do so much and trust me when I say that we are already putting you first.

A case of selective amnesia

The case I am going to tell you about in this chapter is a typical example of how the ED is that place where we are expected to solve any problem, regardless of whether it is a medical issue or not.

It is the start of a night shift. The nurse in charge comes to ask me to 'please see this patient whose wife is making a fuss' about having to wait. Remember what I said in my previous book about being seen quicker the louder you shout? Well, another example of how that behaviour is rewarded.

Reluctantly I grab the patient's notes and, while slowly walking to the cubicle, I read what the triage nurse has written. *32-year-old male, money missing from bank account after a business trip to Amsterdam. Wife thinks he was drugged and robbed.* My first impression is that a) this is not a medical problem, never mind an emergency problem, and b) this is the advanced version of *my drink has been spiked*. I enter the cubicle.

The story goes as follows: the patient went to Amsterdam on a business trip 3 days ago. While in Amsterdam, his card was used to withdraw £2k from his bank account, and he denies any knowledge of how this happened. His card was not stolen, his wife is showing it to me, and it has not been used again since the said £2k withdrawal 3 days ago. Therefore, the wife's working theory is that her husband was drugged and forced to withdraw the money from his account. But of course, the husband, a.k.a. the patient, has no recollection of this ever happening. He is just sitting there, looking like a little lamb that is being taken to the slaughterhouse. The wife does not seem to find it odd that, should her theory be valid, the perpetrators might as well have taken all the money in the account while her husband was drugged, or the card and pin code and withdrawn as much money as possible as fast as the cash point allowed them to. Yet, this did not happen. The wife brings the patient to the ED to have a full battery of drug tests to support her theory. Can you see the emergency yet? Neither can I. This is clearly, if anything, a case for the police. Although I have my own suspicions, I prudently do not propose any alternative theories, but rather explain that this is not a medical issue, that we do not do drug testing, and that if she is concerned, she should speak to the police. She, of course, is not happy with my plan, and so reluctantly takes her husband with her, the poor sod thinking *this is not going to end well.*

On an additional note, the husband had not cancelled the card or informed the bank, because I am pretty sure they would request CCTV camera footage from the cash point used to withdraw the 2 grand in Amsterdam and, in his amnesia, he probably has flashes of himself in the company of a couple of prostitutes. If the image resolution is good enough, it might even show some white powder around his nostrils.

Conversations that never happened between a doctor (D) and a patient (P)

Male in his 20s. Attends for injury to left wrist 3 days ago while on holiday in Greece.

D: Did you see a doctor in Greece?
P: Nope. I didn't have travel insurance and they wanted to charge me 150 euros for the consultation alone.
D: The x-ray does not show any fractures, but I suspect a scaphoid fracture. These fractures typically do not show on early x-rays but do after a week or 10 days. I will apply a futuro splint, you know, one of those velcro splints, and refer you to fracture clinic for them to x-ray you again in a week.
P: Fracture clinic? Will it be with Mr Winston?
D: I really couldn't tell you who will be doing the clinic the day of your appointment.
P: I'd rather not see Mr Winston. I had an injury to my knee 4 years ago and he was useless.
D: What do you mean by that?

P: He didn't do anything, even though I kept coming back with pain.
D: Did he just do an x-ray and send you away?
P: No, he arranged several x-rays which came back normal, an MRI which didn't show anything, and after a few follow up appointments referred me to physio, which didn't do any good either.
D: Well, I am not taking any sides here, but it looks to me like Mr Winston did everything to investigate the cause and manage your pain, but found nothing to treat.
P: He was useless.
D: Maybe you should go back to fucking Greece and get it investigated there then.

Male in his late teens, brought in to the ED by ambulance in the early hours with testicular pain of sudden onset.

D: I have examined you and I cannot find anything wrong with your testicles. Take some painkillers at home and see how it goes.
P: How am I getting home?
D: You will have to make your own way.
P: But there are no buses running at this time and I have no money on me. I have left my wallet at home.
D: I am afraid there is not much I can do about that.
P: The ambulance brought me here. Had they told me I would have to go back by taxi, I would have brought my wallet with me.
D: You can always pay for your taxi when you get home.
P: But I have no cash, just a debit card.
D: You can pay the taxi with your debit card.
P: But I have no money in my account until I get paid next week.
D: Please get out of my fucking sight.

Girl aged 4, brought in by her mother after a fall. Initially limping but given painkillers in ED and now child is running around and climbing onto chairs happily.

D: So everything seems to be fine now.
P: I am really worried because she was limping earlier and that is not normal for my daughter.
D: I am sure she has hurt herself, but that doesn't mean that she has broken or dislocated a bone or a joint. Besides, she is running around normally now.
P: Yes but I am really worried because she was limping earlier and said that it really hurt. Can you not give her an x-ray just to make sure?
D: Don't you think if I tell you that, in my professional opinion, which by the way is what you came here seeking, your child has not broken or dislocated anything, I am making a clinical diagnosis, saving your child unnecessary radiation and taking responsibility for it?
P: Yes, but I am still really worried.
D: And you think I am not worried? Do you really think that I want to put my job, my reputation and my registration on the line? The easy thing for me to do is to x-ray everything, but I have to protect my patients from unnecessary harmful radiation.
P: Could you still give her an x-ray?
D: I am sorry but this is not a buffet where you chose what you want and you get it. In my professional opinion, as a qualified physician with years of experience, an x-ray would do more harm than good, therefore I am not going to request one.
P: But...
D: Very well, I will sign for one, but as there is no indication for it, you will have to pay for it, in advance.
P: How much does an x-ray cost?
D: £110.
P: Thank you doctor for being able to rule out a fracture without an x-ray.
D: I thought you were really worried.
P: I feel much more reassured now.

Woman in her 30s with some bullshit pain in her belly for 3 months.

D: The good news is that there is nothing of concern.
P: Are you sure?
D: (Fuck no. I want you to go home and die.)
P: The last time I came to hospital I had to push for an x-ray, because the doctor was not very good.
D: Why did you think you needed an x-ray?
P: I don't know, I am not a doctor.
D: And did the x-ray show anything?
P: It came back normal.
D: So the doctor that was not very good didn't want to do an x-ray because he knew it would be normal, and you, admitting that you are not a doctor and know fuck all about x-rays, pushed for an x-ray that didn't show any abnormality.
P: Yes.
D: You are a fucking idiot of the worst kind.

20-year-old female accompanied by her mother (M), already with a cast on her left arm for a recent fracture, has fallen onto her right hand and the x-ray shows a broken right wrist requiring another cast.

M: How is my daughter going to cope? She lives on her own.
D: Perhaps you could look after her, since you are her mother.
M: Could she not be admitted to hospital?
D: What. For a month until the fractures are healed?
M: Yes.
D: The hospital is overwhelmed with patients to the point that there are not enough beds and you want your young and healthy daughter, who obviously has at least you to help her, to block a bed for several weeks?

M: She cannot cope so you need to do something.
D: Maybe it is you who needs to do something. Why do I, or the NHS, have more responsibility towards your daughter than yourself? Aren't you her mother?
M: Yes but it is your responsibility.
D: I would say it is *your* responsibility. And your demands are purely selfish. So you would want to take nurses away from the ill and elderly to attend to your daughter? Your. Daughter. What about if we admit her but we charge her, or you, the cost of the bed, £400 per day, multiplied by 28 days... £11,200. How does that sound?
M: I'll take her home. We'll sort something out.

Woman with a twisted ankle.

P: I missed a step and twisted my ankle. I can walk on it but it hurts.
D: Have you taken any painkillers?
P: No, I didn't want to mask the symptoms.
D: Please fuck off home, take some painkillers and if your ankle still hurts disproportionately, then come back.

Man with a hand injury and a history of a missed fracture years ago.

D: Your x-ray has confirmed that there are no broken bones in your hand.
P: I don't trust you. You guys have missed a fracture before.
D: What do you mean you don't trust me? It wasn't me who missed your fracture. And what do you mean by "you guys have missed a fracture before"? We are not cells in a multicellular organism. We are individuals, so you cannot blame me for someone else's mistakes. A patient once stole my mobile phone and I don't treat you as if you were a phone thief. We don't even refer to patients as "those guys." The fact

that a patient is rude or a time waster does not mean you guys are all the same.

P: I still don't trust this hospital.

D: Well, you obviously do, since you are here. People don't go again to where they have had a bad service. Do you take your car to the garage that ripped you off? Or go for a meal to that restaurant that had shit service? There are more than 1000 hospitals in Great Britain, yet you came to this one. So stop the crap and get the fuck out of my sight.

Suicidal threats and overdoses

In the 5th Century BC, the Greek writer and geographer Herodotus, considered by many as *the father of history*, once wrote: "When life is so burdensome, death has become for man a sought-after refuge." The threat of suicide, or the suicidal intent, is not something to be taken lightly. When someone is in such a metaphorical deep dark pit that the only perceived way out is ending one's own life, that someone deserves to be treated with the utmost empathy and care. However, working in the ED, a place like no other to develop cynicism, we start peeling layers of concern when people talk about suicide with a smile on their faces. And this, I am afraid to say, has become the norm. A person that successfully kills himself does not attempt it multiple times before they finally achieve their intended goal. We literally don't see them in the department. They do it, and they make sure they are going to succeed, often to the shock of those close to them, who did not see such a tragic end coming.

What we more often than not see in the ED is so called suicidal intents seeking either attention or personal benefit. Patients will threaten with jumping in front of a bus, for such extremely serious situations as not being granted a paid taxi home, not being given the painkiller of their choice, often opioids, and other similar demands. I can give you several examples: a woman that demanded a taxi home after being discharged to be able to feed her cats, threatening with hanging herself if her request for a paid ride home was not granted, which makes you want to ask her who the fuck is going to feed her fucking cats if she kills herself?; a middle aged man, intoxicated and shouting that he was going to kill himself, even asking medical staff to help him end his life, developing chest pain while in the department and then being really scared of dying, to the point of pathetically asking medical staff to not let him die (in this particular case, the thing to do would've been to tell him "There you go mate, your wishes are going to be granted" before leaving him alone in the cubicle); a frequent attender with overdoses, who always tells a friend after she has done it, caught taking even more pills while in the ED, which happens to be the safest of places to not die of an overdose; a teenager brought in by her mother after taking an overdose, and telling me all about it with a smile on her face, as if this was something she did day in and day out, who also happened to develop anaphylaxis (a life threatening allergic reaction) to ibuprofen, so she overdoses on paracetamol instead, just to be safe. I would seriously have more respect for that teenager if she actually licked an ibuprofen and ended up in hospital with anaphylaxis, rather than avoiding the one drug, as easy to buy in a supermarket as paracetamol, that can actually kill her. I hope you get my point.

We also frequently have attenders that have taken an overdose because they wanted to "end it all", but also called the police to tell them what they had done, but insisted that they asked them not come to save them. If not the police, they always tell a friend because, of course, the friend is just going to reply "Thanks for letting me know, mate. I'll book the day off work for your funeral" and carry on watching Coronation Street. Their whole argument is that they did not call the ambulance themselves, so surely, in their head, that makes it more serious.

We also have overdosers who attend voluntarily but once in the department try to do a runner, well knowing that if they go, we will have to search for them and inform the police; self-harmers, who bang their heads against walls, floors, or anything hard, brought to the department after calling an ambulance themselves, to continue doing the same in the ED. We get security to restrain them, and they threaten us with suing for assault. Do you want our fucking help or not? If you don't, why did you call an ambulance? And if you do, stop being such a twat.

If you ask me, these people are idiots of the worst kind. First, because they show no respect whatsoever for those people that are genuinely really struggling and cannot see any other way out. Second, because it decreases the level of concern that we, medical professionals, should have towards legit suicidal patients. There are only so many times you can take someone seriously when they work so hard to demonstrate that they are really taking the piss. And third, because we have to divert a great deal of manpower, which by the way we cannot afford to in an already busy department, with patients that need to be seen, whose waiting times and frustration are increasing, and who are going to, on top of that, put us at the receiving end of their dissatisfaction.

The funny thing about all this is that none of those regular "suicidal" attenders ever actually commit suicide. Believe me, they've been at it for years. People die from crossing the road, from a head injury after slipping on a banana peel, from being in the wrong place at the wrong time, even from falling downstairs in their own houses. And yet, these people that claim to be making an active effort to kill themselves seem to have more lives than a fucking cat. When reviewed by the Mental Health team, they are always discharged, and if they are discharged it means that there is no concern about them actually going through with it. Am I sounding quite cynical? Yes I am, but this is what dealing with people that have access to an ED any time of the day or night for whatever reason, medical or not, repeatedly does to you. And not only to doctors. We get a new receptionist and within a few weeks, they join the Cynics' Club.

You are probably thinking that what I am saying is out of order, but let me leave you with a thought I mentioned earlier in the Prologue chapter: at the beginning of the pandemic, the EDs were a pleasure to work in. Only patients that actually needed to be here were here:

no time wasters, no minor complaints, not even, and this is my point, people attending with overdoses. How do you explain that a supposed mental health issue suddenly stops happening in an unprecedented time of uncertainty and fear? The anxiety levels should go through the roof. Instead, they actually got better, if we measure them in terms of mental health related attendances, suicide attempts or even actual suicides. A study published on the 20th of April 2021 in the Lancet, one of the most prestigious medical journals in the world, did not find any increase in suicide rates from the time the lockdowns began nor in the months after the easing of lockdowns. So, clearly the overdosers were not overdosing at that time. My theory is that those frequent overdosers now didn't take overdoses because they knew they would have to attend the ED, their usual place of safety, where they could catch a virus that they thought could actually kill them, and that was never their real intention. Without the safety of the hospital available, as usual, they were abstaining from actually taking overdoses. That, again, should speak for itself, and perhaps be considered when the time comes to implement some changes.

Where the Sun don't shine

In my previous book I purposely avoided mentioning the usual topic of patients attending the ED with objects stuck in their rectums. This seems to be a matter of great interest to people I meet when they find out I am an emergency physician. The 2 questions I usually get, and this is probably extended to my Emergency Medicine colleagues too, are: what is the worst thing you have ever seen, and how many objects have you removed from people's anuses? In that order. So I did not want to use the cliché. However, after reading an article published in the Daily Mail with the headline *Britons cost the NHS £350,000 every year by shoving beer bottles, deodorant cans and toothbrushes in their rectums, study reveals*, I could not stop myself from dedicating a chapter to it.

If you think the cost of these incidents to the NHS is outrageous, let me tell you about the people that I have seen coming to the ED requesting post-exposure prophylaxis (PEP) treatment after having sex with a prostitute resulting in a broken condom, or after having unprotected sex with a stranger on a drunken night. The cost of PEP is somewhere between £600-900 for a regular 1-month regime. And that is just one person being treated. So if these people are entitled to expensive treatment, who are we to criticise those who insert things in their bums because it costs the NHS money?

I have seen over the years people, I mean adults, swallowing objects that I thought were unswallowable, such as mattress springs, needles, batteries of all shapes, and razors. How the hell can anyone gulp stuff like that when some people can't even swallow a paracetamol? I have also seen a patient that inserted a whole ball pen into his urethra that I had to actually squeeze, or milk, if you will, out. I have had to remove a forgotten tampon that did not stop the patient from having sex with it deep inside her vagina nor her partner from showering it with his loads for the several weeks it took this woman to realise that something really stunk down there.

Then I have seen quite a few objects inserted into rectums, from kinder eggs full of drugs to vibrators in full action and dildos made of rubber, plastic and glass. I know, glass, classy hey? However, I have not seen a pattern in terms of gender or age. Perhaps I wasn't paying attention to minute details like that: an object in the rectum is an object in the rectum, whether that rectum belongs to a pensioner that got a bit adventurous or to a teenager exploring his or her sexuality. And that is why I found the mentioned article most amusing. Fun facts I have learnt from reading it:

- An average of "400 objects are removed from English anuses every year" costing the NHS, which is to say you and me, £340,000 per year, or around £850 per object. These figures are set to increase and include immigrants too.
- It is suspected by the researchers that gave us those enlightening figures that people feel inspired by internet porn thus inserting into their rectums anything they can get their hands on. No specific internet porn site was mentioned as a possible culprit, in case you are asking for a friend.
- 85% of the objects that needed to be removed were in male rectums. 1 in 6 of those rectums was at least 60 years old, and I would add, therefore full of haemorrhoids.
- The Chief Executive of the thinktank *Taxpayers Alliance*, dropping a pearl of wisdom, told the Mail Online "Of course accidents happen". I would add that accidents can also happen several times per month affecting the same rectum.

- At least the advice given is top class: "To play safe, please use an object with a flared base to prevent it from getting lost inside". So there you go, no cucumbers or courgettes. Definitely no carrots either. Use instead a dildo with massive rubber bollocks.

While doing some research to write this chapter, I came across quite a few Freedom of Information requests to several Trusts across the UK where the questions were a) the number of operations the trust had done to remove rectal foreign bodies (FBs), b) what FBs, and c) how these FBs were disposed of once removed. I have a sneaky suspicion that these requests were made by people who want their FBs back. The responses, however, were quite amusing and varied. It turns out that some Trusts do not keep a record of the objects removed, while others classify them quite accurately as "deodorant", "carrot", "metal bar", "bottle" or even "pen", with "vibrator" being by far the most preferred object used to stick up one's own arse. Contrary to popular belief, hamsters or toy cars were not listed amongst those FBs. All Trusts admitted to not having a defined protocol or guideline as to what to do with the FBs once removed from the patients' rectums, since those FBs could not only be the consequence of a sexual experiment gone wrong, but also the result of a violent attack or even drug mules caught on duty, and therefore those needed to be handed over to the Police. Nowhere was there any mentioning of whether they had a specific protocol for washing the FBs before submitting them as evidence. The Wye Valley NHS Trust specifies that what happens to the FBs after removal is "dependent on the nature of the foreign object and the circumstance around how it entered the body." However, the Royal Stoke University Hospital's answer to that specific question about disposing of the FBs was: "The object is disposed of or handed back to the patient depending upon what the object is and the wishes of the patient." Aren't they nice? You want your dildo back so you can stick it up your arse again? Here you go my friend. Please leave us a good review. Also, if you needed to, now you know where to go for the best service.

An extreme case of rectal foreign bodies, so extreme that it made it into a publication in a medical journal in 1986, is the case of a 20-year-old man whose boyfriend injected cement mix through a funnel into his rectum, followed by a ping-pong ball to aid retention. I really don't know what they did that for, or what they were expecting to happen next, but lo and behold the cement mix solidified, the pain started and, unable to pass it naturally, the man ended up in hospital, where the surgeons managed to remove the FB, a perfect mould of the man's rectum, without causing him any damage. Kudos to them. I would've loved to be the ED doctor attending this case just to hear the explanation of how the cement got in there. It would definitely be of particular interest, in this case, to find out what happened to the solidified cement rectal mould with an embedded ping-pong ball as a finishing touch, whether it was given back to the patient to take home and use as bespoke ornament, or whether it ended up in a surgical museum. If you do an internet search, you can find pictures of it. If you find the x-ray, you can even see the ping-pong ball.

Darwin Awards are given to, basically, stupid people that attempt something really stupid and die in the attempt. Now, in order to qualify for a Darwin Award, a person must remove himself from the gene pool via an "astounding misapplication of judgment." I looked up their webpage and I was pleasantly surprised that they had awards presented to people who had inserted stuff in their rectums. There were a few interesting ones:

- A man who treated his constipation by inserting a live eel in his rectum. Why he thought this would help is still under investigation. The eel had started eating the man's colon, perforating it and causing peritonitis. Luckily for him, surgeons were able to remove the animal and save the man's life. I do believe that these types of incidents help to advance surgical science. Not a true awardee in the sense that he did not die in the attempt, but the level of stupidity well deserved at least an honorary mention.

- An alcoholic who due to a painful throat ailment decided to insert 3 litres of sherry up his ass and ended up dying. A true award winner.
- A female inmate that smuggled an automatic pistol into a high-security prison who ended up having to have it removed surgically and survived. Who would've thought a vagina does not make for a good gun holster?

I have not witnessed this yet, but it is only a matter of time before someone with a perforated appendix is shouting "Where is the on-call surgeon? I am dying in here" to be told "Shut up, she is busy removing a massive dildo from someone's arse!"

As a side note, during my research, I also found "How to remove object from anus at home" to be a popular search sentence in Google, and I was moved by the amount of good people out there giving good advice on the subject. It turns out that people with things up their arses do not misuse the ED and try whatever they can at home first. Wouldn't it be wonderful if everyone did that for everything else?

Stepping into my shoes (Part 3)

After making sure she is not pregnant, having had a feel at her belly and listening to her heart and chest, it has taken me a great deal of my time to reassure and discharge my patient. She insisted on knowing why her belly hurt. I explained, several times, that we don't always have an answer for why a condition, or a pain occurs. We don't know, just to give a couple of examples, why people suffer from headaches, or even why we do something as contagious as yawning. We only make sure it is nothing that needs treatment here and now, we are emergency physicians after all, so if she is that concerned about her belly pain, she should really make an appointment to see her GP for further management, investigations or whatever it is that GPs do these days. She wanted to have an abdominal CT scan. I explain that a CT scan is not indicated, never mind as an emergency, and that it would expose her to a brutal amount of radiation that she does not require. I have also told her, as you may have noticed I do a lot, that the easy thing for any doctor is to full body CT scan everybody, but we have a duty to protect them from tests that can result in harm. She doesn't seem to give a shit about what I think (what do I know about emergency medicine, after all?), so to let me know that she is grateful for how much I care about her health, she has reminded me that she will sue me if I am wrong and happen to miss something, and I have told her that that is perfectly fine but to please send me a thank you card if I don't and I happen to be right, letting me know what an amazing doctor I am. I take her to the exit and tell her to have a lovely day, but what I really want to tell her is to fuck off. I hope it is becoming clear to you, my dear reader, that no one cares about us: management would not give a rat's arse if we died of exhaustion as long as patients are seen and discharged from the department sausage factory style; our regulatory body, the fucking GMC, contrary to what the regulatory bodies of any other profession or trade do, excluding nursing, which is protect its members, is there to sodomise us at the slightest opportunity and without any type of lubrication; and patients are just vicious and vindictive when it comes to making complaints. I will elaborate more on this matter in the *Stupid things we (still) do* chapter.

 I write the consultation notes, take her off the system and pick the next patient's notes, going again through all the fucking process of finding a cubicle and all that. When I finally have a space, I walk to the WR, but another doctor stops me on my way and asks me if I can give a hand with a difficult canulation. So here we go again: another set of notes that are going on an adventure in the back pocket of my scrubs.

 When I am done using my ninja skills to canulate my colleague's patient, I start making my way to the WR. On the way, a paediatric senior nurse smiles when she sees me. She was looking for a doctor to help in the paediatric area. She's got 2 juniors that apparently are not that confident and are taking their time so she needs someone who can see little patient's faster, reduce the waiting time and decongest the paediatric area of the department. I tell her to give me a couple of minutes to drop the notes off and take my name off the patient I was about to call. After doing this, I arrive in the paediatric department. Nurses' faces light up as they start looking at the notes to let me know who they would like me to see next. I run through the children they are concerned about, and after sorting them out, or at least making a plan for each one of them and initiating some sort of treatment, I pick up the next notes: a perfectly healthy boy who has been brought in by his mother to the ED 13 times during the period of his short 7 months of life. That is more times than many adults in their 50's have attended the ED. Always discharged, never anything wrong found with the child. When I see the name, I think *her again*. We all know this mother. She is a frequent flyer and now that she has a baby, she obviously wants him in the club too. Problematic, never happy with the advice given to her, nor to her child. She has been known to leave the premises escorted by security. The emergency today: her boy is constipated. Not vomiting, not in pain, not showing any signs of a blockage in his intestines or anything, he just has not pooed for 4 days. I know, and everybody else knows, that this is not going to end well. I examine the child while he is there happily kicking his legs and smiling at me, grabbing my stethoscope and doing the normal things that healthy children his age do. I am only examining the child as a way of reassuring the mother, not because I need to check that there might be something wrong with him. Children of that age don't lie, you can tell when they are not happy just by looking at them, and this child was having a great time trying to chew the rubber on my stethoscope. I brace myself to tell the mother that there is nothing of concern for a child that has not pooed in 4 days, to continue feeding him as normal, and to see the GP if the problem persists. As I say every new phrase of advice, I can see her face turning into that expression that I have seen so many times before, which she makes before starting to make counter arguments. "So are you telling me you are going to leave my child like this?", to which I respond "Like what? He is absolutely fine. Look at him." The child seems to be on my side, let's out a fart and kicks all limbs simultaneously while he smiles widely. She then asks if I am absolutely sure that there is nothing wrong with her child. I ask her what she has got in mind, expecting to hear about one of the causes of constipation that Dr Google has to offer, to which she responds "I don't know, I am not a doctor," implying that were she a doctor, automatically she would know what to do. This is my opportunity, "In that case, guess who is a doctor, you stupid twat." I wish we could say that. The "you stupid twat" part of my response only happened in my head, but no need to say she still was not happy and once again, she had to be escorted out by security while she shouted obscenities on her way out. I just smiled and waved her goodbye. With such pleasant customers, how can I not love my job?

Once the paediatrics area is back to normal pace, I have a chat with the nurse in charge, and go back to the adult side. And by this I don't mean the part of the ED where there are shelves full of dildos on display, or where giant screens play porn non-stop. I hope that was understood. On my way back I walk by a cubicle and I recognise that particular smell that the trained nose can identify as the unpleasant scent of a water infection. It is funny how we can diagnose conditions by smells. It is actually a clinical skill that ancient, and not so ancient doctors, were proficient in. We can diagnose a very bad bowel obstruction by the fetid smell of burps or vomit; or a bleed in the stomach by the smell of the stools. A diabetic ulcer has a distinctive sweetish, nonetheless foul odour that permeates through the air of the whole department, invading the fabric of our clothes and lingering in the nose for some time. Death has a similar smell, although not as intense, which can be smelt sometimes on those patients that have not got much time left on this Earth. The worse smell, however, is not any of those I have just described, but that of an abscess caused by anaerobic bacteria, and not just because of the horrid stench, but because it stays in your nose for several days and every fucking thing seems to now smell of it. Taste was also a diagnostic tool for those who set the foundations of medicine for future generations. This way of diagnosing gave the names to the different types of diabetes. Diabetes literally means to pass through, perhaps referring to the increased amount of urine produced by patients affected by the condition, and noticed by ancient doctors to have a sweet taste, or *mellitus* in Greek, meaning honeyed or sweet. It is attributed to the Oxford University physician Thomas Willis, who in 1674, was the first western doctor to connect the sweetness of the urine to the condition suffered by its owner and to add the word *mellitus* to the name of the disease. Diabetes insipidus, on the contrary, is a rare disorder not related to lack of insulin or even to sugar, that causes the body to produce too much urine, but so diluted that it tastes of nothing. As you can guess, the only way ancient doctors had to diagnose which kind of diabetes they were dealing with was to sip the patient's urine from a glass and taste it. When or even why someone even thought of checking the taste of someone else's piss is still a mystery. Luckily for me, we can rely on the biochemistry lab today.

So once I go to the patient's box to get the next patient's notes, the first thing I get is a bollocking from the doctor in charge, passive-aggressively accusing me of having taken a long break. After I explained where I was, and how I have managed to drastically reduce both the number of patients and the waiting time in the Paediatric ED, I am just asked to carry on and see the next patient. No apology or anything. With the amount of bollocking we get coming from all angles, I sometimes wonder how no doctor has as yet flipped, and come to work with a machine gun, Falling Down style, blowing every motherfucker that moves into pieces.

The next patient. I take the next patient's notes. I read the next patient's triage notes and I realise the next patient I am going to see is what we call a *diva patient*. Multiple unexplained symptoms, not related to each other, like for example, itchy scrotum and shortness of breath. Diagnosis: a typical case of bollocks, but I still have to go, take a history, examine the patient, take responsibility for a bollocks condition that is definitely not an emergency condition, and most likely, get some bollocking from a dissatisfied patient when I tell him all of the above, perhaps avoiding saying bollocks so much. At least this patient is already on a trolley, as diva patients usually are, due to their dying duck manner. In my head I start counting how many complaints I have had this month and whether I can afford to have another one. It really beats me to try and understand what these people are thinking of to attend an ED for such bollocks. I get the part where they have noticed something unusual, like shortness of breath, but I cannot even remotely comprehend how they themselves don't notice that a person who is truly struggling to breathe has a feeling of impending doom and cannot even complete a sentence to explain that they are short of breath, while these motherfuckers can talk for England. Anyway, off I go.

I find the cubicle where the patient is and as soon as I introduce myself, the status of diva is confirmed. Sign number one: patient talks to me with his eyes closed and fast tiny contractions of the upper eye lids. Why would anyone do that? Being short of breath does not make you close your eyes, neither does having an itchy scrotum. So why? Sign number two: "I don't know" is the common denominator to all the patient's answers. When did the shortness of breath start? I don't know. When did you notice an itch in your scrotum? I don't know. Hmm, let me lay my hands on your itchy scrotum and feel your energy field, perhaps that might help with making a diagnosis. Do these people take their cars to the garage and say I don't know when asked what the problem is? Do they go to restaurants and instead of ordering food from the menu just say they are hungry? Sign number three: everything hurts. I place the stethoscope on his chest to listen to his heart and it hurts. I ask him to breathe deeply to listen to his lungs, and it hurts. Maybe the itchy scrotum has no testicles inside? Sign number four: new bollocks symptoms are thrown in as the history taking and examination progresses, like having noticed a scratchy feeling in both eyes, or making faces of pain when feeling their bellies. I conclude my examination and my preconceived diagnosis of a clear case of bollocks remains intact. Of course, my diva patient has had blood samples taken on arrival, so now I must wait for those results before being able to discharge him.

You might think that this is an easy patient, and that I should not use the word bollocks so much when referring to his presentation and diagnosis, but this type of patient is inherently noxious, for they turn us into hard-core cynics. They are the ones that stop us from taking genuine patients that present with bizarre symptoms seriously (remember the "there is no never"?) They are comparable to drug seeking attenders, complaining of pain to get a free dose of morphine or benzodiazepines on the NHS. Drug seekers, by the way, are the reason why we think twice before giving strong painkillers to patients with unconvincing pain, for you to understand where I am coming from. There have been cases of youngish people complaining of chest pain, behaving in a dramatic or exaggerated way, that have not been given the attention that they truly needed and, as a result, have ended up suffering harm as no one diagnosed the clot in their lungs that was causing the symptoms. "We thought he was faking it" is a common reflexion in retrospect, and diva patients and the cynicism they originate are to blame for it. Before you explode with indignation and reach conclusions similar to those reached by patients in the WR when I make patients that can walk walk, remember that we are also human, with all the pros and cons that come with it. In the same way that we are deeply affected by tragedies, to the point that our profession has a high suicide and addiction rate, we also become complacent after years of spending time and effort with people that come repeatedly complaining of symptoms that we thoroughly investigate to find nothing. Over and over again.

More common phrases and complaints

Since writing my earlier book, more of these pearls have been reminded to me in my day-to-day work. So here we go.

I pay your salary/for the NHS with my taxes

Very well, that is an irrefutable truth, if you do indeed work and pay taxes, but let's not forget that I, and everybody that works for the NHS, pay taxes too. The reason why anyone would say this to a doctor or nurse is because they are demanding some sort of preferential treatment, not because they are going to suggest a pay rise.

If we are going to use tax to measure how much treatment one is entitled to, it follows that the opinion of whoever contributes the most should weigh heavier. So considering that the median household disposable income in the UK was £31,400 in the financial year 20/21, and a doctor's wage is well above that average, therefore the tax contribution is much higher, by those standards, the great majority of people who make that kind of idiotic statement should shut the fuck up and fuck off.

I love the NHS

I love the NHS was an expression widely used during the Sars-Cov-2 pandemic, mainly written on posters with rainbows and hearts, celebrating the heroic actions of all of us who came to work to do the job we are paid to do, pandemic or not. I don't even know what it was all about, making us all heroes, clapping for us every Thursday and the rest, only to treat many of our colleagues and other members of staff as disposable when the vaccine mandates were either implemented in the case of Nursing Home staff, or threatened. That's what happens in the military: send people to war with the alleged reason to serve their country, then leave them homeless, jobless and psychologically scarred. We are treated like condoms: absolutely necessary one moment, disposable the next.

Saying *I love the NHS* during a respiratory virus pandemic is like saying *I love toilets* during a norovirus gastroenteritis outbreak. The NHS is not a family business that relies on its customers to survive. We are kind of the opposite. Our real customers, the people that really need us do not choose to come to the ED, but rather have no other choice. Have you ever seen the NHS advertising as if it was McDonalds or Gillette?

So *I love the NHS* is kind of a rhetorical statement, like *I love the atmosphere*, or *I love fresh water*. If we didn't have an NHS, we would be fucked, with no one to treat us, to provide care for us and our loved ones when we need it the most, without having to remortgage our houses to pay for it. So please, save us the crap.

I don't know, I am not a doctor

This is normally said by people who disagree with a treatment or investigation plan, as if the person who is making the diagnosis and/or the treatment plan was not a doctor either. It is also said by those who, when told that before attending the ED it would've been sensible and preferable to try simple things, like taking paracetamol and/or ibuprofen, respond that they don't know if what they have is an emergency or not. Do they sit on the toilet all day because they don't know if they need to poo or not? Do they eat continuously because they don't know if they are hungry? Are they really that stupid? You don't need to be a doctor to know something is really wrong with your body, like you don't need to be a mechanic or know anything about cars to know when something does not sound right in the engine.

The ED is the only service I can think of where we are not allowed to tell people that they should not be here, or that they should take painkillers before attending or that they shouldn't have called an ambulance to then decide to drive to the hospital rather than wait a long time for it to arrive. I don't really understand why we are not allowed to discuss these issues with patients. It would be better for everyone.

I didn't want to mask the symptoms

I really don't know where this idea originated or even why it is perpetuated. No amount of over-the-counter pain killers is going to mask any symptoms that will lead to a misdiagnosis. I don't even understand why people think of treating the pain as masking the symptoms, instead of, well, treating the pain. Allow me to elaborate.

It is very disappointing, and dissatisfying at the same time, witnessing first hand that after a minor injury such as a sprained ankle, or a contusion, the first priority for a considerable number of people is to attend their local ED, as opposed to taking some simple painkillers and seeing what happens, or in the first instance trying to deal with it at home, like people with foreign bodies in their rectums do. It should not be a normal occurrence that people are discharged from an ED with no intervention needed, other than advice or simple painkillers, and yet, according to the NHS, around 9 million people get sent home from A&E every year after receiving only advice at a cost of £1.4 billion. I think we can all agree that an ED's purpose is not to function like a checking and reassuring service, mainly because it takes resources from the people that really need them, not to mention taking the satisfaction out of the job. Parents even do this not-masking-the-symptoms shit with their children. Let me say that slower: parents allow their children to be in pain, something that we would be severely criticised for doing, so their symptoms are vivid and made worse when being examined by the nurse or doctor. So not trying simple things at home before coming to the ED is plain selfish, even neglectful in the case of parents. When you think about it, it is cheaper for a person to attend the ED by ambulance than to take some simple painkillers at home. This is plainly wrong and a system that not only allows, but encourages that practice via 111, is doomed to fail. It would end in a flash if there was a charge for attending. Justifying this behaviour as not wanting to mask the symptoms is plain stupid. Which takes us to the next common phrase:

I just wanted to make sure it's nothing

What the fuck do people mean when they say this? Do they mean they knew it was nothing but wanted a doctor to say so? No one with a serious condition said that. Ever. Yep, my bone was sticking out of my thigh, but I just wanted to make sure it was really broken. My chest felt like an elephant was sitting on it, I was vomiting profusely, sweating like a motherfucker, couldn't breathe, but I just wanted to make sure it was a proper heart attack. To them it might just seem a case of feeling reassured, but for someone in severe pain that has to wait because the doctor is busy reassuring someone else is no laughing matter. This behaviour, once again, would not be a thing if there was a charge for attending the ED.

Stupid things we (still) do

Anyone foreign to the medical profession would think that doctors follow guidelines and protocols, and the expertise of all doctors is kind of the same for the particular field they work in. This is obviously wrong. Think of any other profession; think of the several plumbers, builders, electricians, or lawyers you have met as a customer over the years. Some were good, some were excellent, some should simply change careers and do something else. Medicine, and nursing for that matter, is just the same.

So it follows that some of the things we do, are not supported by current guidelines, or by evidence but rather are based either on the dangerous statement "because we have always done it this way" or on logic that only makes sense to a few and nobody dares to challenge, so it perpetuates itself. Other practices, unfortunately becoming common, are for example the use of Wikipedia by doctors, instead of reputable medical sites, to look up conditions. So there you are, in the ED, waiting to be seen while the doctor that will see you is reading in Wikipedia how to manage your condition. I personally find it unacceptable. If I was being charged with murder, I would not want my lawyer browsing through Wikipedia to prepare my defence, in the same way that I would not want an architect consulting Wikipedia to design my house. I really can't understand the doctors that think looking things up on a website that anyone can edit and is not free of bias is acceptable when dealing with the wellbeing of a patient.

Now, let me tell you a few of the things we do that make no sense. I will have to elaborate for you to understand where I am coming from, like giving medication to someone having a seizure, which to the untrained person might seem like the thing to do, but it is not, actually. So let's start with that one.

Seizures

A seizure happens when there is a sudden, intense burst of electrical activity in the brain. This causes the messages between cells to get mixed up and it can manifest in several ways, depending on the area of the brain involved, but the ones I want to focus on are the generalised tonic-clonic seizures that most people are familiar with. In the vast majority of cases, these seizures are uncomplicated in the sense that they are self-limited, with a maximum duration of 2 minutes. Therefore, no emergency treatment is needed, other than making sure that the person having the seizure does not suffer any further harm as a result of all the kicking and shaking. Rarely, these seizures fail to stop within the expected time; we call this *status epilepticus* and only then treatment is indicated with antiseizure medication, namely, a benzodiazepine, commonly lorazepam. After a seizure, the person enters what we call the post-ictal period, characterised by confusion which slowly improves on its own, typically lasting between 15 to 30 minutes. If we administer a benzodiazepine when we shouldn't, first, it is unnecessary, and second, it prolongs the post-ictal period, and can complicate the return to normal breathing. Every guideline on the subject does not recommend starting such treatment unless the seizure has been ongoing for at least 5 minutes, yet every time someone has a seizure in the ED you can hear someone requesting and even administering lorazepam.

Wheelchair and trolley use

In my previous book I dedicated one whole chapter, titled *On Wheels*, to this topic. Nothing has changed since, so I feel compelled to discuss it again.

As I have mentioned already, the ED is that place where you can go read your book comfortably on a trolley while waiting for your test results. You don't like reading and prefer to spend time on social media? No problemo señor, that option is also included in the package. Paramedics bring any patient, ambulatory or not, on a stretcher or wheelchair. The reason given is that if they fall and hurt themselves while in their care, it is their responsibility. I think this is a misconception of what their duties are, and an exaggerated fear of complaints. That takes us back to what I have repeatedly mentioned regarding everyone being scared of litigation. And at the end of the day, I can't blame them, considering how unprotected staff are in an environment where blaming and punishing is the norm.

So for instance, a person that has fallen 3 days ago and has hurt her neck attends the ED after having been walking around for 3 days. The moment a fractured vertebra is a possibility, that person will be put on a trolley, neck immobilised with blocks, and won't be able to have an x-ray until lying flat, even before any fracture has been diagnosed. The argument is that if anything happens while in our care, it is our responsibility. Never mind that the patient has been walking about for 3 days or even that the patient does not think it is necessary to lay on a trolley for an x-ray. Recent studies have shown that immobilising is not risk free and can cause harm, but as usual, it is one of these cases of "we have always done it this way".

If you want to do the test yourself, next time you go to ED, sit in a wheelchair. I can guarantee that, unless you encounter a doctor like myself, you won't have to take a single step around the department.

Paracetamol overdoses

The whole idea of taking a drug with suicidal intent, is to take lots of tablets of a chemical that will make your heart and breathing slow down, or your blood pressure or blood sugar drop, or liquify your blood so much that it will make your body systems fail and ultimately kill you, just to give a few examples. To start with, if anyone wants to kill themselves, paracetamol should probably be the last drug to attempt it with. People have this weird idea that if you take a lot of anything that can be bought from a chemist, or from the medicine shelf in the supermarket, you go to sleep and never wake up. Paracetamol neither makes you sleep nor stops you from waking up. So if you take a paracetamol overdose and go to sleep, you are likely to wake up at most with abdominal pain and vomiting. A day or 2 later, you will still be vomiting, and your liver will start to fail. On day 4 you start turning yellow, like Homer Simpson yellow, meaning that your liver is fucked, and with it your clotting factors, so you start bleeding. The kidneys might start to fail, and the pancreas might get inflamed giving you pancreatitis, which is, in itself, bloody painful. On day 5, either recovery starts or organs start giving up one after the other, and only then, you might die. As you can see, if you want to kill yourself in a totally awful way, then paracetamol is your drug of choice, although you might want to try rat poison or pesticides for a similarly horrible experience.

For us to decide which paracetamol overdoses we need to treat by administering a drug that will protect the liver from damage, we need 3 pieces of data: when the overdose was taken, how much was taken and the person's weight, since we work in milligrams (mg) of paracetamol per kilogram (Kg) of patient. Current guidelines tell you that if a patient has taken less than a toxic dose, which has been estimated to be 75mg per kg in 24 hours, you don't even need to do any blood tests or check the paracetamol levels, as we know that it is very unlikely that that dose will cause any harm. On the other extreme, if we cannot ascertain with a certain degree of accuracy how much was taken, or at what time, the safest thing to do is to start treatment straight away. If in doubt, treat.

So let's say someone comes to the ED saying that they have taken a certain amount of paracetamol and they tell us the time they did it. We do our calculations and it turns out that it falls in the non-toxic dose category. All we have to do is contact the Mental Health team to review the patient and that is the end of our involvement. Unless you want to make things complicated and not believe the dose given by the patient. Then you do blood tests to check for paracetamol levels. But the levels, to mean anything, have to be considered with the timing of the ingestion, which is the part in which we believe that patient. So we believe that the overdose was taken when the patient says it was taken, but we don't believe the amount that the patient is telling us they've taken. This, I hope you can agree, makes no fucking sense. Either we believe the patient, who after taking an overdose has attended the ED or we don't believe a word the patient says and start treatment with the antidote straight away. Anything in between is bollocks.

Thinking outside the box

You might think that as highly trained and skilled individuals, we would be able to use the box just as a reference, but you could not be more wrong. There are 2 factors to consider here: first is that highly trained does not mean highly intelligent; and second, the usual being forced into submission by those who do not think outside the box. I will give you 2 typical examples:

- The way patients are screened for sepsis. Contrary to popular belief, sepsis is an extreme response to an infection. The immune system goes mental into killing mode and starts attacking everything in sight causing extreme inflammation to the point that it becomes life-threatening. I say contrary to popular belief because the word sepsis has become so mainstream that a chest or urinary infection is referred to by patients and other health professionals as chest or urinary sepsis. As you can imagine, the transition from infection to life-threatening sepsis is a complicated chain reaction triggered by bacterial toxins, resulting in the uncontrolled release of hormones and inflammatory mediators with names as complex as macrophage-derived cytokines. It is important that this reaction is caught early (within what is classically defined as *the golden hour*) and aborted, before everything gets out of control to the point of no return. Instead of teaching staff what sepsis is so they can make sense of presentations, they are given a tick box chart that screens for high or low temperature, fast heart rate, fast respiration and other parameters. If a patient meets any of those criteria, they are given a dose of antibiotics intravenously. The problem is that there are many conditions that are not sepsis and can present with those same symptoms, for instance a viral infection or a severe bleed, but since staff are not properly trained nor understand the physiopathology of sepsis and instead just tick boxes, a huge number of doses of antibiotics are given unnecessarily making it very easy for bacteria to evolve into antibiotic resistant superbugs. So paradoxically, by trying to blanket treat everyone with an infection for sepsis, we are teaching the bacteria that cause sepsis how to beat our antibiotics.

- Non-accidental injuries. To safeguard children, medical and nursing staff are asked to be as vigilant as possible and to look out for a series of presentations suggestive of non-accidental injuries (NAI) as well as whether the account of how it happened is consistent with the injuries and the time frame in which the injuries occurred. For example, a delayed presentation should be considered carefully, as should fractures of long bones, like the thigh bone, or bruises in different stages or on children that cannot mobilise due to their age or other reasons. The aim is that if any of these factors are present, it should make us think of NAI. In reality what happens, surprise surprise, is that if you take your child with a long bone fracture even without delay and with a perfectly consistent mechanism of injury, it will automatically trigger a safeguarding concern. Common sense of the type *have some pain killers and we'll see*, for example on a fall or on a head injury with nothing to suggest the parents should be concerned, is not rewarded, for if you then take your child to the ED the following day, it counts as a delayed presentation, and that makes you a fucking criminal, apparently. It is the equivalent of the police treating the relatives of every 90-year-old that dies at home in their sleep as murder suspects until proven otherwise.

Complaints handling

In any other organisation complaints are a way of identifying flaws in a system, making the management accountable to the public; a feedback mechanism where users can highlight shortcomings, prompts to review both organisational and employees performance and conduct, aimed at action being taken and improvements made. For this, it must be easily accessible, and users must be encouraged to use it if appropriate. A complaints procedure, in any other organisation, is a good thing. When I mentioned earlier that we, NHS and ED staff, are now perceived and treated as supervillains, I extend this also to the complaints we get, which seldom fulfil the intended purpose of improving anything, but are mostly a waste of everybody's time since "The doctor didn't say hello to me" or "The nurse didn't offer me a cup of tea" are not really complaints, are they? It is so ridiculous that people choose not to take any painkillers before coming to hospital and then file a complaint because they were not offered painkillers in the ED.

If you've read my previous book, you will know that when you make a complaint against a doctor, a nurse, a receptionist, an insect that flew buzzing by, or even about the department's decoration, you will receive a response and even an apology letter. There is this thing that angry patients have about asking for names: they always want to know the name of whichever member of staff is involved. I don't see that happening in any other private or public services with such enthusiasm. If a person is not happy about the service provided by the waiter, or the parking attendant, they just make a complaint, or leave without tipping, but they don't routinely ask for the person's name. Our names are attached to the case history, so asking for a name is just a cocky display of perceived authority, that only the NHS allows users to have. Angry customers also shout to us to get out of their sight, to go away, when it is we who are in our place of work. Does anyone go to their bank manager's office, have a dispute about, say, a rejected loan application and tell the bank manager to get out of their own office while they stay in it?

Service users and dissatisfied patients tend to exaggerate their complaints, always adding that the doctor or nurse was rude to them, that they felt intimidated, that they are vulnerable, conveniently omitting details in an attempt to validate their claim. Those that exaggerate, become vicious and want the doctor's registration revoked, their source of income gone, their lives ruined. They can accuse us of anything they like: from having frowned at them to eating new-borns for breakfast, and everything in between, although being rude is the all-time favourite. Being rude, it seems, is not requesting an investigation or not prescribing a treatment that is not indicated in the first place. Demanding that a medical professional acts against their knowledge and expertise is, apparently, not rude at all. The Trust will not only ignore any civil wrong offenses such as defamation, libel or slander, against staff but will also take the complainant's statement as ultimate truth, the burden of proof being left to the member of staff. How's that for being required to always be a respectable and responsible member of society, but being treated like a piece of shit when that should come in handy? It is as if not having that x-ray or that blood test that is not indicated in the first place triggers the forementioned vicious desire to destroy the clinician's life. You might think that I am overstating, but I know a male doctor that was accused by a female patient of touching her inappropriately when examining her ankle, for not arranging the x-ray that she wanted. We can agree that the lower part of the leg is well away from any intimate body part, therefore a doctor would not request the presence of a chaperone to perform such examination. And yet, the accusation was acted upon without any other consideration, the doctor was suspended immediately, referred by the hospital to the GMC who instructed an investigation that lasted months and his professional life was forever ruined. All he was doing was his job, as well as protecting the patient from unnecessary radiation. Another case comes to mind, also related to an x-ray not requested for a patient that demanded having one when it was not indicated. Remember that the clinician does not pay for the x-ray from his or her pocket and will request any examination regardless of how expensive it is, if it is needed. In this case, the patient, made a complaint for not having an investigation that was not indicated, that would've exposed him to unnecessary radiation, that he did not know anything about, and yet the Trust asked the clinician to apologise to the patient. The clinician told the Trust to go fuck themselves. Can you imagine? Doing something in the best interest of a patient and being told to apologise, effectively, for acting in the patient's best interest. Are we fucking crazy? Ladies and gentlemen, this is the state of the NHS.

We have all heard of random people having cardiac arrests in the community, a member of the public happening to be a doctor, providing good Samaritan care, bringing that person back to life only to be sued because cardiac compressions resulted in several broken ribs. Although there is a strong ethical duty on all doctors to help in an emergency, there is no legal obligation, at least in the UK, to do so outside our place of work. However, once a doctor gives assistance, a duty of care is automatically established with all the documentation, consent, standard of care and the rest, including the risk of being sued.

Some countries have even passed legislation to protect doctors in these situations. I personally feel less and less inclined to assist anyone outside my place of work. Sadly, this is the consequence of being fed up with getting complaints even when I have done my very best, which for some reason, it is still not perceived as enough.

On that note, I would like to suggest and ask of you that if you attend your local ED and receive a good service, please spend a few minutes of your time leaving a nice written comment about the members of staff that you have interacted with. A feedback system that only receives complaints and no compliments unfairly reflects badly on our performance in the eyes of management. So if you are unhappy, by all means make a complaint, but if you are satisfied with your experience through the ED, please do something nice and leave a nice comment. It is really no effort for you, it goes a long way in showing that we really care, and it makes our day to see that we are appreciated.

What could you have done better?

Reflection is a big part of what is expected of every medical professional. But there's learning from your mistakes, and then there's the type of absurd reflection we are often expected to do. For example, you own a restaurant, a customer is dissatisfied with how the steak has been cooked, and instead of calling the Maître d' to complain, they start shouting out loud that they asked for the steak to be cooked rare and it is medium rare. You try to calm the customer down, offer an apology but it does not change the situation. Meanwhile, other customers are having their meals disrupted. Having tried everything and having no other choice, you ask the customer to leave but they refuse. Then you call the police to remove the customer from your premises. But your employees side with the customer, and the police, on arrival, does exactly the same. The customer demands that you get out of his sight, and the police, to diffuse the situation, takes you to the kitchen while your staff makes the customer a cup of tea. Then the police ask you to reflect on what you could've done better to have avoided this confrontation. So you have to reflect on it and write it down. You are even supposed to learn a lesson, perhaps attend a course on dealing with dissatisfied customers. I hope you understand the analogy.

Treating friends or family

We are not allowed to treat our own relatives. Each year a significant number of doctors are reported to the GMC, by snitch pharmacists mainly, for prescribing to someone they know. The reason: an emotional attachment is bound to affect our judgement or focus. I personally think this is a load of bollocks. Who is going to treat my children or my partner better than myself? I have tried to find publications with specific evidence about this issue and have found absolutely nothing. I can understand that, if any of us was leading the resuscitation process for one of our friends or relatives who has suffered a cardiac arrest, we would find it difficult to stop the efforts despite how long the resuscitation has been going on for, or how dead our friend or relative looks, because in that particular scenario our judgement will be clouded by our emotions and we will refuse to give up, but what kind of emotional attachment can affect my focus when prescribing antibiotics for my partner's water infection? If I was a surgeon, who would take my daughter's appendix out more carefully than me? To me this is as ridiculous as not allowing a mechanic to repair their own car, or not being able to get your brother, a qualified plumber, to do the plumbing installation in your house. Besides, think of when you have a medical problem, and informally you call your doctor friend for advice. Doesn't that make sense to anyone?

Over-the-counter medications

The next stupidity I would like to discuss is the administration of over-the-counter medication, paracetamol as an example, to patients by nurses. Any idiot can buy paracetamol in any supermarket or convenience store and administer it to anyone they like; a patient can be dispensed ibuprofen and be told that they can take it every 8 hours, and there is no safety issue with that, but a qualified nurse has to do a special course to independently give paracetamol or ibuprofen to a patient. I even know a case of a nurse who gave ibuprofen to another nurse who was suffering from a headache at work, and because it was not prescribed, she was submitted to a disciplinary procedure, with the subsequent amount of time wasted and paperwork generated along the way. The equivalent of you having a disciplinary procedure for taking home a paper clip from the office.

Paperless

Being paperless is something that Trusts proclaim proudly, as if it was true. You would think that this means that everything is documented and requested on computers, without the need for printers. An x-ray could be ordered, the order sent to the x-ray department, and the x-ray pictures sent back to the computer. In the same way, blood tests could be requested in that manner, transferred electronically to the lab and the request matched to the samples once received. But this is far from being the case. For instance, there are commonly used IT systems in which x-rays are requested on the system, the request printed out and taken to the radiology department only to be scanned by the radiographers. Same applies to blood tests. In every hospital I have worked, there is more paper after being declared paperless than before. Having said that, ordering an x-ray for a female of whatever age opens a prompt window that asks whether this 62-year-old female is pregnant. There is no hope.

Software systems

In England and Wales, every trust has a different software system that does not link with any other Trust's. This usually means that what happens in a hospital is completely inaccessible from any other hospital. You would think that in the age of the internet, if you were visiting another part of the country and needed to go to the ED, or even if you were referred to a specialist unit in a different Trust, the referrer would be able to access updates, changes in medication, test results and the rest, but that couldn't be farther from what happens in reality. I didn't bring my medication because it is all in my records, patients tell us, to our despair. This lack of sharing information is also very favourable for malingerers and drug seekers as, when they are well known in one ED, they just make their way to another, and the staff there have no way of knowing that that particular person has just been given 10mg of morphine iv in the morning, or that they are not supposed to admit that other person because they will invariably steal from the other unsuspecting inpatients. There is no clear reason for this. Every Trust and every GP surgery should be able to use the same software system, connected to a central database, where every patient is identified with an unique number, for instance, their NHS number, and every medical condition, medication and test results accessible from any other Trusts or GP surgeries. There is no need to have a chip implanted with the person's medical history, a centralised database is all that is needed.

Alcohol detox regimes

I will start by saying that there is no way of helping someone who does not want to be helped. Successful detoxification regimes rely on both medical and behavioural support, so it follows that medical therapy alone is useless. That is why addicts have to register with whichever organization operates in their area, join a waiting list mainly to show commitment and carry on drinking as usual until therapy starts. I am not going to bore you with specific details, but we often get people straight from the pub, drunk as a skunk, demanding to be detoxed because they cannot carry on like this. Instead of pointing them in the right direction, we admit them, we medicate them, they occupy a bed for several days until they discharge themselves straight back to the pub. It is so predictable that it makes no sense to keep doing the same. Another waste of your tax money.

Stepping into my shoes (Part 4)

My next patient, after discharging the diva, is an 88-year-old female, nursing home resident, known to suffer from Alzheimer's disease, that terrible illness that not only takes away our ability to form new memories, but also digs holes in our minds, extirpating brutally what is left of our dignity, and of the person we once were. She suffers also from a myriad of illnesses for which she is administered daily a copious amount of medication, to keep her alive and prolong her agony for as long as possible. There is no proof of this, but I believe people with dementia are in a permanent state of suffering due to the constant disorientation. It must be like that feeling of entering a room and not remembering what we went there for, or being spoken to by someone that seems to know us, even hold us dear, but we haven't the faintest idea of who they are. Imagine feeling that 24/7. They are not alone in their anguish for it expands inevitably, although for different reasons, to their loved ones as well. As I walk to the cubicle where she is being nursed, I remember having seen her shouting for help, trying to get off the trolley, her hospital gown twisted, exposing her naked body for all to see. As I arrive, I notice that there is no carer accompanying this patient and the triage notes are very vague, with a very poor handover from the paramedic crew, so I have no idea of why this patient has been brought to the ED.

I look at her next of kin information only to find that she has no next of kin. Poor soul, I think while my heart melts. She is all alone in this world, with no one to care, and I mean properly care for her best interests, not just feed her, dress her and put her to bed. Before I call the nursing home for information about whatever it is they've sent her to us for, I approach her to see how far she can communicate. She is laying on her left side, legs tangled in the trolley's railings, on her quest to break free. I call her name, Elsie, as she likes to be called, her real name being Margaret, and she freezes. Slowly turns her head towards me and the draft of a smile is drawn on her lips, as if she was trying to respond. Her eyes shine no light, but a deep void, whatever is left when hope is gone. She looks at me, scrutinising, as if searching for a memory that will reveal to her who I am, but she finds none, so she turns again to the task in hand. I put my hand on her shoulder, but I get no response. She's started to whisper something and I lower myself to hear what she is saying. "Mommy, mommy," she is calling to no one. Alone in this world, she calls for her long dead mother, trying to regain her primordial feeling of safety as a child. Feeling my eyes fill with tears (how embarrassing), I walk to the station to find a phone and talk to someone at the nursing home. I see her nurse going into the cubicle with an HCA to get her cleaned and changed.

It turns out that they called the GP for a routine visit, since Elsie seemed a bit more confused than usual, however you measure that. They sent a GP paramedic who, for reasons that perhaps only the GP paramedic understands, performed an ECG and found "some changes", the usual and quite common trick to deflect responsibility onto someone else. I look at the ECG and see nothing of concern for a patient of this age.

All Elsie needed was perhaps some antibiotics to cover her for a water infection and to be reviewed in a few days' time with a simple telephone call. Instead, she is sent to the ED, an unfamiliar environment well known to cause distress in patients with dementia, stripping whatever still remains of her dignity on the way. Not to mention the extra burden on the ED, which by the way, cannot offer any more than what I have just mentioned. We live in a world where no one knows what they are doing any more, where no one is prepared to take any responsibility, where although the mantra is *whatever is best for the patient*, the reality is that there is no heart. The GP paramedic thought he or she could not take the responsibility for a patient that was not clear cut, so made up some bullshit excuse about ECG changes, something that even if true, would be completely unrelated to her being more confused, and dumped her onto the ED. A common occurrence. As annoying and heartless as it sounds.

At this point, Elsie has been cannulated and blood samples have been sent to the lab. Not because there was an indication for them, but for the reasons I explained in my previous book. After my examination and reviewing of the results I cannot find anything of concern. I, however, start her on antibiotics, just in case. Orally, nothing fancy. I ask her if she would like a cup of tea, and I make her one, little milk, no sugar. Amazing how her brain still remembers how she likes her cups of tea. I transfer it to a cup with a beaker, so she cannot spill it and burn herself. The expression on her face, her smile when I brought her the tea, that made my day. Forget about all the cunts I've had to deal with today. Forget about everything. Seeing her smile made it all worth it. She seems to know how to drink from that, she is used to it. Good. I speak to the nursing home to send her to her own room and bed, but they are reluctant to take her back until the morning. Hospital transport is massively delayed due to the overwhelming number of patients that are waiting for a ride home, and Elsie is not likely to be back until past midnight. Nursing home policy, to avoid disturbing other patients when they are asleep, is not to accept anyone back after 9 at night. It makes sense, I guess, to avoid the risk of waking up other residents with Alzheimer's and trigger a chain reaction of chaos in the rooms and corridors in the middle of the night. Elsie will have to endure another few hours of fear and disorientation for something that could've easily been dealt with at the nursing home. If the person sent to the home instead of the GP to review her could've given a shit.

My shift is nearly finished. I make sure all my documentation is done, my cases closed, and I have let one of the night doctors know about Elsie. After prescribing her night and morning medications, I make my way to her to make sure she is comfortable. She is still laying on her side, no longer struggling to break free. I look at her for a little while, while I remind myself that she is alone in this cruel world. She must have sensed my presence, because she turns onto her back and looks at me. I ask her if she is ok, and she extends her arms, reaches out to me with a smile. Maybe she wants to sit up, so I take her arms to help her, but she pulls me towards her, still wearing a smile, and hugs me. She does not utter a word, just keeps hugging me. I hug her back, for I don't know how long, until she lets go. That might be the only hug she has had in a long time. My eyes are flooded with tears. As she lets go, she looks me in the eye, briefly frowns, and slowly and peacefully leans back onto her pillow, resting her hands on her chest. She stares at me, smiles and nods, then she closes her eyes. As I come out of the cubicle, I can see faces looking at me, perhaps because I have tears in my eyes, perhaps because they think it was unprofessional to hug a patient. But I don't give a shit. She has brightened my day, although in a bizarre way, since it has done her no good to be taken from the nursing home unnecessarily. Or has it?

The end of my shift, the time to go home. The time I have been waiting for all fucking day. I think back to the times where I used to come to work with excitement, with eagerness, with a smile on my face. I search my memories in an attempt to find when it all changed, but I cannot visualise a precise moment but rather a process of becoming increasingly disappointed. Years of enduring verbal abuse from colleagues and patients alike; of trying to do my best to help people and being criticised for it, even having to answer vicious complaints from those I went the extra mile for, as apparently, an extra mile was not enough. Years of asking for favours to get my patients x-rayed, or scanned, or made comfortable; years of having to put up with the egos of idiots that probably live miserable lives and find their revenge opportunity at work; years of being crushed into not giving a shit, to be able to fit in and not lose my sanity.

While I get changed, I reflect on the patients I have seen today, and the only one I have actually done anything for that is worth mentioning, is Elsie: a cup of tea and a hug. That is the highlight of my day, the interaction that makes me feel remotely like a doctor.

This is not the Emergency Medicine I signed up for. This is not even practicing medicine, but rather dealing with cunts and hypochondriacs. It used to be about proper stuff, cardiac arrests, broken limbs, life threatening infections, people that were in very bad condition after an accident or an injury. People that I could help with medication, with my knowledge and skills. People that were grateful for what I did for them. Now I have no idea what most of the patients I see daily are in the department for. It is like people attending because they have yawned, or sneezed, and demanding tests and answers; making complaints because nothing was done about their itchy armpit. The ED is overwhelmed, full of people that have nothing seriously wrong with them, demanding more, reducing us, doctors and nurses, to being mere servants, facilitators of their wishes. I send most of them home with a diagnosis of No Abnormality Found. In the process, I get anger and abuse, lack of respect and bollocks coming from every fucking corner. This is definitely not what I committed my working life to.

I became a doctor because I believed in humanity, because I loved interacting with others and helping those in need at every opportunity. Instead, being a doctor is turning me into this person I never imagined I would become, for whom all hope in altruism is lost. A person that used to run to attend to any emergencies that happened in his path but now looks the other way and cannot give a shit because all he sees is a potential lawsuit. A doctor that is ashamed of telling strangers that he is a doctor when they ask.

This is what working in the NHS had done to me. And I promise you, I used to love my job.

OUTRO

So here is where we are now. The NHS, the one national service that should be defended with all our might, is crumbling. Nothing is more important than a healthy population; nothing more precious than access to free, well, paid through taxation, but you know what I mean, universal healthcare. And we are letting it be demolished in front of our own eyes by the very same people entrusted to look after it. It is time for you to get involved.

Sicko, the 2007 documentary by Michael Moore, should be watched by everyone in the UK and certainly by anyone living in a country with a National Health Service. It is about how private healthcare in the USA is a heartless beast that favours doctors that decline expensive treatments, even if their decisions have fatal outcomes for the insured. It depicts real cases to give examples of the financial burden of being diagnosed with cancer or a chronic disease and not having health insurance. People with fingers accidentally amputated at work having to choose which ones they can afford to have reattached, the price of the cheaper finger being $12,000; couples in their retirement age becoming homeless after being forced to sell everything to pay for their chemotherapy. It is obviously very biased, but it gives a good idea of what it means to not have an NHS.

We, the healthcare staff, have tried, but have failed miserably. You see, it is difficult to keep fighting the good fight when everything and everyone is against us. We are tired. Tired of not being listened to by the cunts in charge that could both, improve the service and make our lives better along the way. Tired of only being noticed when something goes wrong. Tired of the same people, regular attenders, system parasites, presenting with nothing, but pretending to have fits, or strokes or belly pains, over and over and over and over again, using resources, taking our time and diverting it from the people that really need us. Tired of having to answer to these twats' written complaints demanding even more care instead of them using the system appropriately and going through the right channels. Tired of putting up with the bullying that the posters on the wall claim will not be tolerated. Tired of being verbally abused, sometimes even physically assaulted, and all of it being brushed under the carpet. Tired of having to ask for favours to get our patients x-rayed, or made comfortable, as if it was for our own personal benefit. Tired of pointing out flaws and being told to shut the fuck up. Tired of going home exhausted, wondering why we do this in the first place. In a sentence, tired of doing the impossible for the ungrateful.

So the ball is in your court now. Yours is the fight. Those politicians and patients and managers responsible for the crumbling of the NHS are actively working to destroy it. Politicians, because they probably have private health insurance and corporate friends ready to get a slice of the cake when the NHS is privatised in exchange for [insert favour here]. Patients, because they are selfish idiots that are only concerned about themselves. Managers, because their thing is quantity and not quality. Always focused on how many patients are waiting, and bollocking doctors and nurses if those patients are not discharged within 4 hours. They don't care whether it was a safe discharge or if the ward Mrs Goodenough was sent to was the right place for her. The quality of the care patients receive is of no importance to them, their job is to make the numbers look good, without the responsibility, of course, of someone suffering harm, that is for doctors and nurses, who will be severely blamed for their incompetence should the shit hit the fan due to the anally retentive eagerness of managers to get rid of people. They work as if in a sausage factory, but the NHS is not a factory and patients are not sausages, in case that wasn't clear.

If you do nothing, they are bound to win. So please, like I have asked of you earlier in this book, get involved, because your healthcare, and the healthcare of those you love, depends on it. You deserve quality healthcare, by professionals that enjoy what they are doing, that are paid decently and feel they make a difference. You deserve to be looked after with dignity and privacy, not in the middle of a corridor. You deserve to feel safe in hospital, and not threatened by aggressive cunts with violent behaviour patterns that go on repeatedly and unchallenged. When you are poorly and you need to go to hospital, you deserve the best quality care.

Create local groups physically or through social media; write to your local hospital's CEO; invite doctors and nurses, the front-line members of staff that work in your hospital, to meet up with you. Learn from them the journey from registration to discharge, whether admission is needed or not, and discuss the challenges along the way. They work there so they will know how to overcome them, and you can then use that information to work with the Trust on the implementation of changes. Get involved in staff wellbeing, patient dignity and right to privacy, unnecessary bed blocking, hospital transport hours, abusers of the system.

Use the Freedom of Information Act to enquire about how much of your tax money is being spent on taxis for people that are fully able bodied. Ask what is done to identify hard workers, good professionals, and make sure they don't leave. Discuss issues like difficult regular attenders, and how to get them the help they need; violent behaviour and a warning system to actually ban people from hospitals to protect other attenders as well as NHS workers.

Engage with your GP Practice, explore the appointment problem with them. Write to the GMC and ask what they are really doing, other than sitting comfortably in their High Castle offices shouting "Off with their heads!", to ensure their regulations and guidance are being followed to protect healthcare workers and guarantee patient's safety. Write to the RCEM to enquire about how they make sure their guidance is followed to ensure quality care. The RCEM has published a document with the hashtag #ResuscitateEmergencyCare full of recommendations like "expand and retain the Emergency Medicine workforce", "tackling overcrowding" and, basically, invest more money. All very nice but recommending is one thing and knowing what is stopping the recommendations from being implemented is another. You cannot retain workers when the working conditions are shit and staff feel neither protected nor valued. You cannot avoid overcrowding when most users, even managers, don't know the difference between a GP and an Emergency Doctor, therefore people attend the ED with minor complaints as, with its 24/7 open door policy, it's the path of least resistance. Perhaps I, or you, should send them copies of my books.

Write to the CQC and demand that they do not announce their visits. Involve your local MP, and the local press too. It is doable if you get organised. Only then you will see a change for the better.

Printed in Great Britain
by Amazon